S0-DTD-477

DR. M. DAVI

NUTRITION AND FEEDING OF
PRETERM INFANTS

Nutrition and Feeding of Preterm Infants

H.J. Bremer   O.G. Brooke
M. Orzalesi   G. Putet
N.C.R. Raiha   J. Senterre
J.C.L. Shaw

B.A. Wharton
(Chairman)

*Committee on Nutrition of the Preterm Infant,
European Society of Paediatric Gastroenterology
and Nutrition*

BLACKWELL SCIENTIFIC PUBLICATIONS

OXFORD LONDON EDINBURGH
BOSTON PALO ALTO MELBOURNE

© 1987 by
Blackwell Scientific Publications
Editorial offices:
Osney Mead, Oxford OX2 0EL
  (*Orders*: Tel. 0865 240201)
8 John Street, London WC1N 2ES
23 Ainslie Place, Edinburgh EH3 6AJ
52 Beacon Street, Boston
  Massachusetts 02108, USA
667 Lytton Avenue, Palo Alto
  California 94301, USA
107 Barry Street, Carlton
  Victoria 3053, Australia

All rights reserved. No part of this publication
may be reproduced, stored in a retrieval
system, or transmitted, in any form or by any
means, electronic, mechanical, photocopying,
recording or otherwise without the prior
permission of the copyright owner

First published 1987

Printed in Great Britain by
Redwood Burn Limited,
Trowbridge, Wiltshire

DISTRIBUTORS

USA
  Year Book Medical Publishers
  35 East Wacker Drive
  Chicago, Illinois 60601
  (*Orders*: Tel. 312 726-9733)

Canada
  The C.V. Mosby Company
  5240 Finch Avenue East,
  Scarborough, Ontario
  (*Orders*: Tel. 416-298-1588)

Australia
  Blackwell Scientific Publications
  (Australia) Pty Ltd
  107 Barry Street,
  Carlton, Victoria 3053
  (*Orders*: Tel. (03) 347 0300)

British Library
Cataloguing in Publication Data

Nutrition and feeding of preterm infants.
  1. Infants——Nutrition
  I. Bremer, H.J. II. Wharton, B.A.
  613.2′0880542 RJ216

ISBN 0-632-01696-5

Contents

Contributors

Hans J. Bremer, *Professor of Paediatrics, Medizinische Einrichtungen der Universität Düsseldorf, Kinderklinik und Poliklinik, Moorenstrasse 5, 4000 Düsseldorf 1, West Germany.*

Oliver G. Brooke, *Formerly Professor of Child Health, St George's Hospital Medical School, 49 Rusholme Road, London SW15 3LF, United Kingdom.*

Marcello Orzalesi, *Professor and Head of the Departments of Child Health and Neonatology, University of Sassari Medical School, Sassari, Italy.*

Guy Putet, *Practicien Hopitalier, Service de Neonatologie, Hopital Eduard-Herriot, Place D'Arsonval 69374, Lyon cedex 08, France.*

Niels C.H. Räihä, *Professor of Paediatrics and Chairman, Department of Paediatrics, University of Lund, 214 01 Malmo, Sweden.*

Jacques Senterre, *Professor of Neonatology, State University of Liège, Division of Neonatology, Hopital de la Citadelle, 4000 Liège, Belgium.*

Jonathan C.L. Shaw, *Consultant Neonatologist, Department of Paediatrics, Faculty of Clinical Sciences, University College London, The Rayne Insitute, University Street, London WC1E 6JJ, United Kingdom.*

Brian Wharton, *Consultant Paediatrician, Sorrento Maternity Hospital, Wake Green Road, Birmingham B13 9HE, United Kingdom.*

Preface

The European Society of Paediatric Gastroenterology and Nutrition (ESPGAN) has published three reports on infant nutrition since 1977. This monograph continues the series. The eight authors were appointed by the Society to issue guidelines on the nutrition of the preterm baby. We held 15 meetings from 1981 to 1986. Preliminary findings were presented at the annual meeting of the Society in Graz in 1983 and the final document was discussed at the annual meeting in Edinburgh in 1986.

Some of the Committee meetings were held in association with scientific symposia concerning perinatal nutrition to which the members contributed and the proceedings of some of these symposia have been published. The expenses of the Committee meetings were funded from various sources including the associated scientific symposia, the Society, and grants from infant food manufacturers, including Bristol Myers, Farley Health Products, Findus, Mellin, Milupa, Nestle, Nutricia/Cow and Gate, Semper and Wyeth. Without this generous support the work of the Committee and the production of this report would have been impossible.

In spite of all the new data becoming available it has not been easy to formulate a single set of nutritional requirements for all low birth weight infants. Therefore, we felt it necessary to discuss, in detail, the background to, and the reasons for the guidelines. As a result, this report is much bigger than the previous ones published by the Society and so it is published as this book. A supplement to Acta Paediatrica Scandinavica containing only the guidelines will also be published.

Naturally, some recommendations in this book were unanimously supported while others are a compromise view. The recommendations as a whole, however, are the collective responsibility of all the authors.

Brian Wharton,
Belbroughton, UK

Foreword

The survival of low birth weight (LBW) infants, particularly that of very low birth weight (VLBW) infants, has improved dramatically over the past decade. The experience at Babies Hospital (Presbyterian Hospital) in New York is similar to that of other major centres throughout the developed world. At this institution, the survival rate of all LBW infants has increased from 88.5% in 1976 to 94.5% in 1985 and the survival rate of VLBW infants, (i.e. those weighing < 1250 g at birth) has increased from 59% in 1976 to 88.5% in 1985. Since the number of premature births has not changed appreciably over this time, more prematurely-born infants obviously are surviving now than a decade ago.

The survival of more prematurely-born infants coupled with the expectation that treatments now being evaluated (i.e. intratracheal surfactant therapy) will even further improve survival has refocused the attention of many neonatologists away from attempts to further improve survival of LBW infants by improvements in such areas as ventilatory support towards attempts to improve nutritional management. This, in turn, highlights the many problems encountered in nutritional management of LBW infants. On one hand, the endogenous nutrient stores of prematurely-born infants are severely limited, i.e. it has been estimated that the endogenous nutrient stores of the 1000 g infant are sufficient to permit survival for only about four days without provision of exogenous nutrients. Yet, because of immature and/or unco-ordinated sucking and swallowing mechanisms, poor intestinal motility as well as immaturity of other digestive and absorption mechanisms, these infants usually cannot be fed in the same way as larger, more mature infants. Thus, during the early neonatal period, exogenous nutrients usually must be delivered parenterally or by a variety of enteral feeding tubes.

Assuming that delivery problems can be overcome, an even greater problem emerges: what should be infused into the various catheters and tubes? This problem arises from the lack of clear guidelines and/or goals for nutritional management of LBW infants of any size. This lack of guidelines and/or goals, in turn, creates considerable concern and controversy. For example, human milk, which most authorities accept as the appropriate feeding for term infants, may not be appropriate for infants who are born prior to deposition of the relatively larger amounts of nutrients that occurs, *in utero*, during the last trimester of gestation. In fact, it is reasonably easy to demonstrate that the amounts of many nutrients delivered by reasonable volumes of human milk (i.e. protein, sodium, calcium and phosphorus), even if completely absorbed, are insufficient to permit deposition of these nutrients at intrauterine rates. On the other hand, many believe that human milk contains non-nutritional components that may be beneficial in promoting development of a number of physiological mechanisms and that failure to provide human milk, regardless of its probable nutritional inadequacy, may be detrimental to other aspects of development.

The European Society for Pediatric Gastroenterology and Nutrition is to be commended on their decision to step into this void and attempt to bring some order on it. This volume, the result of the Society's effort, contains few absolute solutions for the many outstanding problems; on the other hand, most have been addressed. The available information pertaining to these problems has been summarized and, based on this information, conservative recommendations have been made. Most important, these recommendations are not simply opinions. The authors of the various chapters have put aside personal opinions and prejudices and have arrived at recommendations based on scholarly consideration of the world's literature concerning the LBW infant's requirement for each nutrient.

In my opinion, this volume represents the most complete compilation of available information concerning nutritional management of LBW infants. It should be extremely useful for anyone who is interested in either the overall problem of nutritional management of LBW infants or a specific aspect of this general area.

William C. Heird, MD
Associate Professor of Pediatrics
College of Physicians & Surgeons of
Columbia University
630 W. 168th Street
New York, NY 10032

1
Introduction

In 1977 the European Society of Paediatric Gastroenterology and Nutrition (ESPGAN) published *Recommendations for the Composition of an Adapted Formula*(1). This was the first of a series of monographs on infant nutrition, and subsequently two others were published — *Recommendations for Composition of Follow up Formula and Beikost*(2), and *Recommendations for Infant Feeding*(3). The purpose of these reports was to provide up to date guidelines for the feeding of normal infants. They were formulated by a committee of experts working in the field, who were assembled under the auspices of an independent and international scientific society. This book continues the series.

Recent advances in the care of low birth weight infants has led to the survival of increasing numbers of very immature infants. The challenge that feeding these babies has presented to paediatricians has resulted in research that has made important contributions to our understanding of their nutrition, and of the role it plays in their immediate survival after birth, and subsequent growth and development. However, in spite of all the new data becoming available it is not at all easy to formulate a single set of nutritional requirements for all low birth weight infants, because unlike term infants, they may have a fivefold range of body weight and a corresponding variation in their level of maturity. Thus the requirements of, for example sodium, may be determined more by the maturity of the kidney than body weight or rate of growth. Because of this we have felt it necessary to discuss in detail the background to, and the reasons for our guidelines. As a result the full document contained in this volume is much bigger than the previous ones published by the society, so the shorter Guidelines are published separately as a supplement to *Acta Paediatrica Scandinavica*(4).

The report is in three sections. This first section (Chapter 1) is introductory. It describes the background to the report, the foods presently available for low birth weight babies, the views of other groups, the methods of assessment available and our approach to the individual nutrients. Section two considers each nutrient in turn and summarizes the conclusions in guidelines (Chapters 2–14). The third tries to translate these guidelines into practical

1

policies for feeding the low birth weight baby, dealing in particular with the use of breast milk, the use of formula, and methods of feeding (Chapters 15–19).

OTHER REPORTS

In the past decade a number of other reports have been published by various national and international bodies concerning the nutritional requirements of newborn infants and the composition of infant formulas for those who are not breast fed. They have been largely concerned with the normal infant and his food. In general their recommendations for the suckling infant were that (a) breast feeding is the most suitable method and breast milk the most suitable food for the young infant, and (b) young infants who are not breast fed should receive an 'infant formula' whose composition is closer to that of breast milk than that of cow's milk. The recommendations of some of these reports have been compared(5,6) but a comprehensive review of them all is not available. The recommendations for the composition of infant formulas are broadly similar but there is considerable variation in detail, for example, in the type of carbohydrate and fat which may be included, and the recommended trace element concentrations. Three reports from national bodies, two from the American Academy of Pediatrics(7,8) and one from the Canadian Paediatric Society(9) have dealt specifically with the requirements of the low birth weight baby. These are useful but brief, and have not given detailed reasons for the recommendations. They are summarized in Table 1.1.

Table 1.1. Summary of recommendations and comments concerning nutrition of low birth weight infants.

Nutrient and units		American Academy of Pediatrics 1985	Canadian Paediatric Society 1981
Energy	kcal/kg/day	Approx. 120	110–150
	kcal/100 ml	Up to 81	Up to 81
Protein	g/kg/day	2.5–5	
	g/100 kcal	2.25–4.5	2.5–4
			Unmodified cows milk protein and soya protein should not be used.
Fat	% of total energy	40–50	40–50
Linoleic acid % of total energy		3	3
		Fat not too saturated or too unsaturated	Caution in use of MCT formulas

Table 1.1 (Contd.)

Nutrient and units	American Academy of Pediatrics 1985	Canadian Paediatric Society 1981
Sodium	2.5–8 mmol/kg/day	3 mmol/100 kcal
Potassium	2–3 mmol/kg/day	—
Magnesium mg/100 kcal	—	6
Manganese mg/100 kcal	5 as in normal formula	—
Zinc μg/100 kcal	500 as in normal formula	500
Calcium	200–250 mg/kg/day	130–150 mg per day
Phosphorus	110–125 mg/kg/day	As potassium or sodium phosphate 50 mg/kg/day if receiving breast milk
Copper μg/100 kcal	90	90
Fluoride μg/day	—	250 if low concentration in water
Iron	Possibly 2 mg–3 mg/kg/day from 2 weeks with Vitamin E. Same dose from 2000 g if receiving breast milk. Insufficient evidence for increased amounts.	—
Iodine μg/100 kcal	5	—
Vitamin E	0.7 iu per 100 kcal and 1.0 iu per g linoleic acid plus 5 iu per day	25 iu per day
Vitamin K	At least 1 mg at birth	—
Folic acid	50 μg per day	50 μg per day
Other Vitamins	Multivitamin supplement providing recommended dietary allowances for normal infants, e.g. Vitamin D 10 μg; Vitamin C 35 mg; plus amounts in a formula	Multivitamin drops, e.g. Abidec, PolyVisol
Other comments	Calorie intakes of about 120 kcal/kg/day in formula volumes of 150 ml/kg/day will support the desired weight gain in most infants.	The milk of a mother who gave birth prematurely meets most of her infants' requirements when given at 180–200 ml/kg except for calcium, phosphorus, sodium. Many questions need to be answered before pooled human milk can be shown to be safe and of sufficient nutritional superiority to warrant the cost of establishing milk banks.

NOTE: In many instances the Committees did not give a firm recommendation but quoted results from individual studies, perhaps to be used as guidelines.

4

Chapter 1

AVAILABLE FOODS

Breast milk

Many low birth weight babies receive breast milk either from their own mothers or from donors. The results of a recent and well conducted study of the composition of mature breast milk (supplemented with data from other sources) are given in Table 1.2(10–14). However, breast milk does not have a uniform composition. The concentration of many nutrients changes in the course of lactation, and the milk of mothers of preterm infants may have a significantly higher concentration of protein and sodium than the milk of mothers of term infants. In practice the composition of breast milk received by preterm infants is not known for certain as it is affected by the stage of lactation, the method and time of collection (i.e. drip or expressed milk, fore or hind milk), the mode of sterilization, and the method of storage and administration. Consequently if care is not taken in the collection and handling of breast milk the nutritional quality can suffer (see Chapter 16).

Infant formulas

One of the advantages of formulas is that their composition is known and should not vary. The three major modifications of cow's milk used in the manufacture of infant formulas are the addition of carbohydrate, the complete or partial replacement of the fat by a blend of vegetable and animal fats, and the use of demineralized whey(6,15,16). Low birth weight babies are often given formulas designed for normal babies. Table 1.2 shows the composition of two representative formulas available in Europe and designed for normal babies. It has not been possible to give a comprehensive list of all formulas on the market because there are so many of them and their composition changes from time to time. Also formulas with the same name, but marketed in different countries, may have different compositions.

Other infant formulas have been specifically designed for the low birth weight baby(17) and Table 1.2 gives details of their composition. Energy concentration is usually greater than that of either breast milk or formulas for full term babies. At present all of them are based on demineralized whey; all contain lactose and most contain maltodextrin as well. Fat blends vary, particularly in the amount of medium chain triglyceride (C8-C10) added, which ranges from 0–50%. Mineral content is also variable, for example, sodium concentrations vary fourfold and the stated calcium:phosphorus ratio almost twofold.

METHODS OF ASSESSMENT

There is a wealth of empirical observations concerning nutrition of low birth weight babies on various dietary regimens. Comparison of results from well controlled trials is easy, but further evaluation and the decision 'which is better for the baby?' is difficult and depends on which performance criteria are used in assessment. Should the low birth weight baby mimic the growth of the fetus *in utero* and its chemical development (in terms of body composition and plasma concentrations of various nutrients), or should he be more like the normal breast-fed baby during the early months of postnatal life? Similarly, there are problems with other performance criteria used. For example, balance study errors all exaggerate apparent retention(18), and growth velocity is usually rapid which affects the interpretation of many biochemical measurements of nutritional status(19). Small but statistically significant differences in nutritional measurements may not be biologically important. In clinical practice weight gain is the most commonly used measure of performance, but does not reveal the changes in body composition which occur during growth.

The authors had the general purpose of determining, as far as is possible from the assessment data, the best way to feed low birth weight infants. Under this general heading we have considered the requirements for individual nutrients, the optimum ratio of nutrients to one another, the place of breast milk in preterm infant feeding, and the use of special formulas and supplements. In all these aspects it has been necessary to consider carefully the methods of assessment and evaluation that have been used in the source references. These can be divided broadly into Reference Standards for Growth, Body Composition and Other Methods of Assessment.

Intrauterine growth as a reference standard for the growth of the preterm infant

The principal use of these measures are:
1 to enable differences between *in utero* and postnatal weight gain and chemical growth to be identified and evaluated (recognizing, however, that such differences may not be harmful to health).
2 to enable us to determine whether substances are present in great excess or in inadequate amounts in the diet, by comparing the amounts provided in breast milk or infant formulas with the intrauterine accumulation rate.

Weight gain

There have been many studies of the growth of the fetus *in utero* based on the

Table 1.2. Composition of milks and formulas given to preterm babies. (a) Energy and major nutrients

		HUMAN BREAST MILK				
		Expressed at 6 weeks		Drip	Preterm milk per 100 ml	
		per 100 ml	(per 100 kcal)	per 100 ml	7 day	28 day
Total solids	g per 100 mi					
ENERGY	kcal	70			67	70
	kJ	293				
PROTEIN						
Total	g	1.34	1.9	1.0	2.4	1.8
Casein	g	0.4				
Whey Protein	g	0.8				
Taurine	mg	4.8	6.9			
FAT						
Total	g	4.2	6.0	2.2	3.8	4.0
Butter Fat	g	—				
Vegetable Fat	g	—				
MCT	g					
Other Fat	g					
Polyunsaturated Fatty Acid	% total	7.2%				
Fatty Acids C8–C10	% total	1.5%				
Cholesterol	mg	14	20			
Choline	mg	9	13			
Carnitine	mg					
	nmol	590*	840			
CARBOHYDRATE						
Total	g	7.0	10.0			
Lactose	g	7.0	10.0	6.5	6.1	7.0
Maltodextrin	g	—	—			
Glucose	g	—	—			
Amylose	g	—	—			
Other	g	—	—			

Data

Mainly from the following but some individual figures are from other sources:

Breast Milk

expressed breast milk (DHSS 1977)[6].
drip breast milk (Gibbs *et al.* 1977)[7].
preterm milk 7 and 28 days (Gross *et al.* 1980)[8].
  (see also Anderson *et al.* 1981)[9].
preterm B vitamins at 6 to 15 days and 16 to 196 days of mothers delivering at 29–34 weeks gestation (Ford *et al.* 1983)[10].
For values marked * see chapter for individual nutrient.

Table 1.2 (a) (*Contd.*)

INFANT FORMULAS FOR NORMAL BABIES				PRETERM FORMULAS	
Example 1 based on demineralized whey		Example 2 based on skimmed milk		Range observed in available products	
per 100 ml	(per 100 kcal)	per 100 ml	(per 100 kcal)	per 100 ml	(per 100 kcal)
12.6		14		12.5–15.2	
67.6		70		74–81	
283		293		310–339	
1.5	2.2	2.0	2.8	1.4–2.4	1.9–3.0
0.6	0.9	1.2	1.7	0.6–1.0	0.8–1.2
0.9	1.3	0.8	1.1	0.8–1.6	1.1–2.0
				0.0–5.1	0.0–6.4
3.6	5.3	3.5	5.0	3.4–5.0	4.8–6.3
—		2.1	3.0	0.0–2.8	0.0–3.5
2.4	3.6	1.4	2.0	0.5–2.7	0.8–3.7
—		—	—	0.0–1.8	0.0–2.7
1.2	1.8	—	—	0.0–1.4	0.0–2.1
14.5%		11.2%		15–31%	—
3.3%		2.6%		2–50%	—
3.0	4.4			0.7–1.8	0.9–2.5
				5.0–25.0	7.0–33.0
				0.0–1.0	0.0–1.3
7.2	10.7	7.7	11.0	6.3–9.7	7.5–12.6
7.2	10.7	5.7	8.2	2.3–8.7	2.9–11.6
—	—	2.0	2.8	0.0–5.3	0.0–6.5
—	—	—	—	0.0–2.2	0.0–2.9
—	—	—	—		
—	—	—	—		

Formulas

Infant formulas for normal babies: from manufacturers information based on SMA-S26 (UK) and Milumel (Germany).

Preterm formulas: from manufacturers information based on the following selection of 15 formulas:

Alimento Dicofarm, Alprem, Bebelac Prem, Enfamil Prem, Humana O, Osterprem, MEB, Neomil, Nenatal, Novameb, Preaptamil (UK), Pregallia, Prematalac, Similac 24 LBW or Special Care, SMA Low birth weight or Preemie.

8

Chapter 1

Table 1.2. (b) Vitamins and minerals

		HUMAN BREAST MILK				
		Expressed		Drip	Preterm milk per 100 ml	
		per 100 ml	(per 100 kcal)	per 100 ml	6–15 days	16–196 days
VITAMINS						
Retinol	μg	60	86			
Vitamin D	μg	0.01	0.014			
α tocopherol	μg	0.35	0.5			
Vitamin K	μg	1.5	2.1			
Thiamin	μg	16	23		5	9
Riboflavin	μg	31	44		36	27
Nicotinic Acid	μg	230	329		114	210
B_6	μg	6	9		3	6
B_{12}	μg	0.01	0.014		0.05	0.02
Folic Acid	μg	5.2	7.4		2.1	3.1
Pantothenic Acid	μg	260	371		164	230
Biotin	μg	0.8	1.1		0.2	0.5
Inositol	mg					
Vitamin C	mg	3.8	5.4			
MINERALS (Atomic weight)					*7 days*	*28 days*
Sodium	mg	15	22	13	50.6	28.98
(23)	mmol	0.6	0.9	0.6	2.2	1.3
Potassium	mg	60	86	63	69	60
(39)	mmol	1.5	2.2	1.6	1.8	1.6
Chlorine	mg	43	61		88	59
(35)	mmol	1.2	1.8		2.5	1.7
Calcium	mg	35	50	28	25	22
(40)	mmol	0.9	1.3	0.7	0.6	0.5
Magnesium	mg	2.8	4	2.9	3.1	2.5
(24)	mmol	0.12	0.17	0.12	0.13	0.1
Phosphorus	mg	15	21		14	14
(31)	mmol	0.03	0.05		0.45	0.46
Iron	μg	76	109			
(56)	μmol	1.4	1.9			
Copper	μg	39	56		78★	63★
(64)	μmol	0.61	0.87		1.21	0.98
Zinc	μg	295	421		475★	392★
(65)	μmol	4.5	6.5		7.3	6.0
Manganese	μg	2.0	2.8			
(55)	μmol	0.04	0.06			
Selenium	μg	2–3	2.8–4.3			
(79)	μmol	0.03–0.04	0.04–0.05			
Iodine	μg	7	10			
(127)	μmol	0.06	0.08			
Fluorine	μg	5–30	7–43			
(19)	μmol	0.03–1.6	0.4–2.3			
Chromium	ng	340–430★				
(52)	nmol	6.5–8.3				
Molybdenum	μg	0.5–25				
(96)	μmol	0.005–0.26				

Table 1.2 (b) (*Contd.*)

INFANT FORMULAS FOR NORMAL BABIES				PRETERM FORMULAS	
Example 1 based on demineralized whey		Example 2 based on skimmed milk		Range observed in available products	
per 100 ml	(per 100 kcal)	per 100 ml	(per 100 kcal)	per 100 ml	(per 100 kcal)
79	100	50	72	0.55–150	78–200
1.1	1.6	—	—	0.0–8.0	0.0–10.0
638	943	1400	2000	800–10 000	1000–12 500
5.8	8.6	—	—	0.0–7.0	0.0–9.0
71	105	40	50	37–100	48–135
105	155	50	70	70–500	100–620
528	781	170	240	210–2400	270–3000
42	62	17	24	23–200	30–250
0.11	0.16	0.04	0.05	0.1–0.5	0.2–0.6
5.3	7.8	4.2	6.0	5.0–50	4.4–63
210	311	200	300	250–1500	316–1850
1.5	2.2	—	—	0.0–30	0.0–37
				3.0–130	4.0–171
5.8	8.6	6.0	8.3	10–30	9.0–40
15	22	24	34.3	17–60	24–76
0.7	1.0	1.0	1.5	0.7–2.6	1.0–3.3
56	83	70	99	60–100	76–120
1.4	2.1	1.8	2.5	1.5–2.4	1.9–3.0
37	55	46	66	28–80	37–101
1.1	1.6	1.3	1.9	0.8–2.3	1.1–2.9
44	66	56	80	50–144	67–178
1.1	1.2	1.4	2.0	1.3–3.6	1.7–4.5
5.3	7.8	6.3	9.0	5.0–15	7.0–20
0.22	0.33	0.26	0.38	0.2–0.6	0.3–0.8
33	49	46	65.7	31–72	44–89
1.1	1.6	1.5	2.1	1.0–2.3	1.4–2.9
1270	1880	500	700	40–1300	50–1600
22.7	33.6	9.0	12.5	0.7–23.2	0.9–28.6
50	74	42	60	10–200	13–247
0.78	1.2	0.65	0.94	0.2–3.1	0.2–3.9
370	547	600	850	100–1200	150–1250
5.7	8.4	9.2	13	1.5–15.3	2.3–19.2
15.8	23.4	7.6	10.8	3.0–21	4.0–26
0.3	0.4	0.14	0.2	0.1–0.4	0.1–0.5
		—			
		—			
6.9	10	7.3	10.3	4.0–20	5.0–26
0.05	0.08	0.06	0.08	0.0–0.02	0.0–0.02
10–20	14–29	—	—		
0.05–1.1	0.7–1.5	—	—		

weights of live born preterm infants born at different periods of gestation in different parts of the world(20). Four will be referred to here as most of the reports are in quite close agreement. During the last trimester of pregnancy the growth curve of the fetus *in utero* is sigmoid and can be described by logistic equations describing inhibited growth(21). However, these equations can be approximated by an exponential model of uninhibited growth until growth rate declines at about 36 weeks of gestation. Comparison of estimates of the specific growth rate of the fetus *in utero* obtained by exponential analysis of growth data between 24 and 36 weeks gestation is given in Table 1.3.

Table 1.3. Specific growth rate for fetus' growing along different percentiles (g/kg/day)

Author	10th%ile	50th%ile	90th%ile
Lubchenko *et al.*(22)	15.6	14.4	12.6
Kloosterman(23)	16.6	16.1	14.7
Babson *et al.*(24)	18.9	16.0	13.9
Keen & Pearce(25)	18.0	16.1	15.3

These results are for the most part in very close agreement and the slightly lower growth rates of the infants born in Denver Colorado(22) might be due to the higher altitude above sea level. It seems from these data that since the infants growing along the 10th centile have a faster specific growth rate than the infants growing along the 90th centile, they may have a correspondingly higher nutritional requirement when expressed per kilogram body weight and day. However, the possible implication of this for the feeding of the low birth weight infant has not been explored.

Figure 1.1 depicts the growth chart of a 27 week gestation preterm infant to illustrate the difference between the growth of the fetus and the growth of the preterm infant. Following birth, weight is lost, and there is a delay until weight gain is resumed. Although the weight loss consists of loss of both ECF and soft tissue, the loss of ECF is approximately 78% of the total weight loss(26,27). This disproportionately large loss of ECF in the first week of life results in a change in the hydration coefficient of the body, and the ECF:ICF ratio comes to resemble more closely that of a full term baby. When growth is resumed the ECF volume seems not to return to intrauterine levels and so it is not to be expected that the infant would grow along his intrauterine centile nor that he should necessarily grow at the same rate. However, as in the figure, there is often little difference between the slope of the intrauterine curve and the slope of the postnatal curve and consequently many infants resume their former position on the centile chart without catch-up growth. In others the rate of postnatal growth is less than the intrauterine rate and catch-up growth is

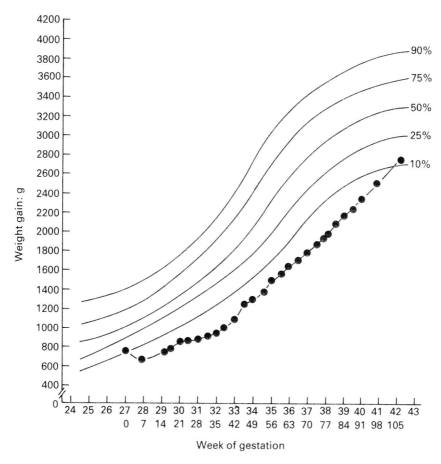

Fig. 1.1. Comparison of the postnatal weight gain of a 27 week gestation infant with the interuterine growth curves of Lubchenko *et al* (1963) (18). The infant resumed her position on the percentile chart without the necessity for catch-up growth.

necessary if they are to attain their former position on the centile chart. It is known that certain tissues, notably bone, develop quite differently in the preterm infant compared with the fetus(28,29) so that even if a preterm infant gains weight at a rate comparable to his intrauterine weight gain, in some respects at least his body composition will differ from that of a full term baby. Indeed because of the change in the volume of the ECF it is uncertain precisely how the postnatal weight gain should be compared to the intrauterine weight gain. Nevertheless when determining the nutritional needs of a growing child it is useful to have in mind a rate of weight gain appropriate to the child's size and stage of development. The specific growth rates given in the table should provide a guide. While recognizing the limitations of these estimates, when applied to preterm infants, we believe them to be valuable, because they emphasize that growth is not linear but a function of mass, and justify us in recommending nutritional requirements on a body weight basis over a wide range of body size even though the 'ideal' absolute weight gain varies from 7.0 g/day for an infant of 500 g to 30.0 g/day for a 2000 g baby. If on the contrary we had assumed that growth was linear (say 25 g/day) we would be recommending nutrients in excess for small babies and in insufficient quantities for large babies.

Chemical composition of the fetus as a guide to nutritional requirements

In each section reference is made to the intrauterine accumulation rate of the individual nutrient where the data is available. These are estimates that have been calculated from the results available in the literature of chemical analyses of fetal bodies. The calculations have been done in a variety of ways(30–32), but all of the estimates suffer from shortcomings, either from including babies whose gestation was not certain or from omitting recent analyses. However, no great precision has ever been claimed for these estimates, and they will surely be improved as more data become available. They are included because they provide a useful guide to the amounts of substances that might be retained in a normally growing preterm infant if he grew at an intrauterine rate. They also draw attention to the very big differences between the intrauterine accumulation rate of some elements and the amounts provided in breast milk and formulas designed for full term infants (e.g. iron, calcium and phosphorus). Such differences do not necessarily result in deficiency but make it much more probable.

Correction of the differences between intrauterine and postnatal growth

In the case of iron, calcium and phosphorus, there will be large differences between intrauterine and postnatal accumulation rates if preterm infants are fed breast milk. Though iron deficiency will develop unless they are given supplements, iron deficiency can easily be prevented by dietary means, because ferrous iron is readily absorbed. With other nutrients, for example calcium, the difference between the amount retained postnatally and the intrauterine accumulation rate is more difficult to correct. On theoretical grounds one can arrive at an optimal intake by dividing the *in utero* accumulation rate by the fractional coefficient of absorption. This, however, results in such a high concentration of calcium and phosphorus in the milk that it is difficult to avoid precipitation of insoluble calcium phosphate, and it is not even clear that such large amounts are either necessary or safe. We do not at present think it wise, by increasing the concentration of nutrients in the diet, to attempt to make premature babies retain all nutrients in amounts equivalent to those laid down in the fetus *in utero*. For example, increasing calcium intake to the theoretical levels would only be desirable if the intestine could tolerate the increased quantity, if calcium absorption was increased, and if the absorbed calcium was actually laid down in bone and not in an ectopic site such as the kidney or aortic valve. Sometimes a benefit may be shown following the administration of a nutrient, for example the effect of vitamin E on the haemoglobin concentration. The benefit, however, may not be considered sufficiently big to make it worth the expense and trouble to supplement all infants routinely. However, it is obviously necessary to increase the intake of a nutrient if a deficiency is likely to occur.

Other methods of assessing nutrient requirements

There are various other methods available for assessing nutritional requirements. Metabolic balance studies can be performed to measure the absorption and retention of different nutrients and the results can then be compared to the intrauterine accumulation rates. A search for the pathological features of deficiency can be undertaken. This has proved a valuable approach in the case of iron, vitamin D, vitamin E, and essential fatty acids. However, in the case of the trace metals copper and zinc though the late effects of severe deficiency are easy enough to detect, the early stages are not. In such circumstances it is often valuable to try the effect of supplementation with a nutrient to see if it may be growth limiting, but unless the studies are very well controlled for other variables the results can be disappointingly difficult to interpret. Often overlooked is the evaluation of adventitious gain of nutrients, for example the presence of trace metals in i.v. solutions or iron in blood transfusions. Equally important may be the adventitious loss of nutrients, for example the loss of iron in venesections or other insensible or unmeasured losses (e.g. in gastric aspirate).

APPROACH TO INDIVIDUAL NUTRIENTS

Each nutrient is considered in a broadly similar fashion under four headings:

Nutritional background

This describes the biochemistry and physiology of the nutrient in the fetus and low birth weight baby. It covers the *in utero* accumulation rate, the consequences of deficiency and excess, and what is known about absorption, retention and insensible losses.

Available foods

This section deals in some detail with the concentration of the nutrient in breast milk and formulas and the factors that affect its concentration, some of which have been summarized above in the section on breast milk.

Requirements and advisable intakes

In this section the reasons for the recommendations are argued in some detail, and the recommendations of other bodies are summarized.

Guidelines

In this section the recommendations are summarized. They are an amalgam based largely on the scientific evidence together with a measure of empirical practice, and where there has been genuine doubt we have erred on the side of caution.

METHODS OF EXPRESSING RECOMMENDATIONS CONCERNING FEED COMPOSITION

Concentration per 100 ml

Milk or formula is in practice measured out by volume and the amount given to an infant is determined by his postnatal age and body weight. It is, therefore, usual for feeds to be prescribed as vol/kg per day. The amount of a nutrient being given to the infant can easily be calculated by the product of concentration × volume. Concentration per unit volume will, therefore, be the most valuable figure for most clinicians. This approach also recognizes that water is the most important nutrient.

Concentration per 100 kcal

This concerns a relationship that cannot easily be varied at the bedside. However, in spite of the relative inconvenience for the clinician of expressing nutrients in terms of energy intake, the method recognizes the interrelations between the requirements of various nutrients and the relatively large proportion of energy used for growth by the rapidly growing newborn baby.

For the normal infant ESPGAN(1), Codex Alimentarius(33), French legislation(34) and the draft EEC directive(35) all express formula composition per unit energy (e.g. g/100 kcal). The British recommendations(36) alone express them per unit volume as fed (e.g. g/100 ml). These differences are of little consequence when considering the normal baby since the energy density of milk and formula fall within a limited range, generally 65–70 kcal/100 ml. However, low birth weight babies may receive feeds with a greater range of energy density (e.g. 65–85 kcal/100 ml) and also receive a greater energy intake, so that the problem of how to express recommendations becomes more complex.

We have decided to express requirements primarily in terms of energy, and have included requirements per kg/day and concentration per 100 ml where it seems appropriate. In Chapter 17 the relationship between volume of intake, nutrient content of a formula and nutrient intake by the baby are considered in detail.

REFERENCES

1. ESPGAN Committee on Nutrition: Guidelines on Infant Nutrition (1977). I. Recommendation for the composition of an adapted formula. *Acta Paediatr. Scand.* (Suppl.) **262**, 1–20.
2. ESPGAN Committee on Nutrition (1981). Recommendations for the composition of follow-up formula and Beikost. *Acta Paediatr. Scand.* (Suppl.) **287**, 1–25.
3. ESPGAN Committee on Nutrition (1982). Recommendations for infant feeding. *Acta Paediatr. Scand.* (Suppl.) **302**, 1–30.
4. ESPGAN Committee on the Nutrition of the Preterm Infant (1987). *Acta Paediatr. Scand.* (Suppl.), in press.
5. Mettler A.E. (1982). Infant formula. In: *Food for the Suckling.* (ed. B.A. Wharton). *Acta Paediatr. Scand.* (Suppl.) **229**, 58–76.
6. Wharton B.A. (1984). Infant formulae. *Bull. Brit. Nutr. Found.* **9**, 83–93.
7. American Academy of Pediatrics: Committee on Nutrition (1977). Nutritional needs of low birth weight infants. *Pediatrics* **60**, 519–30.
8. American Academy of Pediatrics: Committee on Nutrition (1985). Nutritional needs of low birth weight infants. *Pediatrics* **75**, 976–86.
9. Canadian Paediatric Society: Committee on Nutrition (1981). Feeding the low birth weight infant. *Can. Med. Assoc. J.* **124**, 1301–11.
10. DHSS (1977). *The Composition of Mature Human Milk.* Report on Health and Social Subjects No. 12. HMSO, London.
11. Ford J.E., Zechalko A., Murphy J. & Brooke O.G. (1983). Comparison of the B vitamin composition of milk from mothers of preterm and term babies. *Arch. Dis. Child.* **58**, 367–72.
12. Gibbs J.A.H., Fisher C., Bhattacharya S., Goddard P. & Baum J.D. (1977). Drip breast milk: its composition, collection and pasteurisation. *Early Hum. Dev.* **1**, 227–45.
13. Gross S.J., David R.J. & Bauman L. (1980). Nutritional composition of milk produced by mothers delivering preterm. *J. Pediatr.* **96**, 641–4.
14. Anderson G.H., Atkinson S.A. & Bryan M.H. (1981). Energy and macronutrient content of human milk during early lactation from mothers giving birth prematurely and at term. *Am. J. Clin. Nutr.* **34**, 258–65.

15. Wharton B.A. & Berger H.M. (1976). Bottle feeding. *Brit. Med. J.* **1**, 1326–9.

16. Gurr M.I. (1981). Human and artificial milks for infant feeding. *J. Dairy Res.* **48**, 519–54.

17. Brady M.S., Rickard K.A., Ernst J.A., Schreiner R.L. & Lemonds J.A. (1982). Formulas and human milk for premature infants: a review and update. *J. Am. Diet. Assoc.* **81**, 547–55.

18. Fomon S.J. & Owen G.M. (1962). Comment on metabolic balance studies as a method of estimating body composition of infants. With special consideration of nitrogen balance studies. *Pediatrics* **29**, 495–9.

19. Scott P.H., Berger H.M. & Wharton B.A. (1985). Growth velocity and plasma amino acids in the newborn. *Pediatr. Res.* **5**, 446–50.

20. Wharton B.A. & Dunn P.M. (1985). Perinatal growth: the quest for an international standard for reference. *Acta Paediatr. Scand.* (Suppl.) **319**, 1–187.

21. Bonds D.R., Mwape B., Kumar S. & Gabbe S.G. (1984). Human fetal weight and placental weight growth curves: A mathematical analysis from a population at sea level. *Biol. Neonat.* **45**, 261–74.

22. Lubchenko L.O., Hansman C., Dressler M. & Boyd E. (1963). Intrauterine growth as estimated from live born birth weight data at 24 to 42 weeks of gestation. *Pediatrics* **32**, 793–800.

23. Kloosterman G.J. (1970). On intrauterine growth. *Int. J. Gynaecol. Obstet.* **8**, 895–912.

24. Babson S.G., Behrman R.E. & Lessel R. (1970). Fetal growth: liveborn birthweights for gestational age of white middle class infants. *Pediatrics* **45**, 937–44.

25. Keen D.V. & Pearse R.G. (1985). Birth weight between 14 and 42 weeks gestation. *Arch Dis. Child.* **60**, 440–6.

26. Hamilton C.M. & Shaw J.C.L. (1984). Changes in sodium and water balance, renal function and aldosterone excretion during the first seven days of life in very low birth weight infants [Abstract]. *Pediatr. Res.* **18**, 91.

27. Wagen A., Okken A., Zweens J. & Zijlstra W.G. (1985). Composition of postnatal weight loss and subsequent weight gain in small for dates newborn infants. *Acta Paediatr. Scand.* **74**, 57–61.

28. Shaw J.C.L. (1976). Evidence for defective skeletal mineralisation in low birthweight infants. The absorption of calcium and fat. *Pediatrics* **57**, 16–25.

29. McIntosh N., Shaw J.C.L. & Taghizadeh A. (1977). Accumulation of nitrogen and collagen in the femur of the human fetus and the effect of premature birth. *Pediatr. Res.* **11**, 1023.

30. Shaw J.C.L. (1973). Parenteral nutrition in the management of sick low birth weight infants. *Pediatr. Clin. N. Am.* **20**, 333–58.

31. Ziegler E.E., O'Donnell A.M., Nelson S.E. & Fomon S.J. (1976). Body composition of the reference fetus. *Growth* **40**, 329–41.

32. Jackson A.A., Shaw J.C.L., Barber A. & Golden M.H.N. (1981). Nitrogen metabolism in preterm infants fed human donor breast milk: The possible essentiality of glycine. *Pediatr. Res.* **15**, 1454–61.

33. Codex Alimentarious Commission (1976). *Recommended International Standards for Foods for Infants and Children.* FAO/WHO publication. CAC/RS 72/74 – 1976.

34. Ministre de L'Agriculture et le Ministre de la Sante (1976). *Journal Officiel de La Republique Francaise* **215**, 5519–20.

35. Rey J., Astier-Dumas M., Fernandes J., Marquadt P., Nordio S., Oppe T.E., Schmidt E., Senterre J. & Wharton B.A. (1983). Reports of the Scientific Committee on Food 14 Series EUR 8752EN. Commission of the European Communities, Luxembourg. pp 9–32.

36. Oppe T.E., Barltrop D., Belton N.R., Christie A.A., Cooke. J.R., Naismith D.J., Paul A.A., Porter J.W.G., Wharton B.A. & Widdowson E.M. (1980). *Artificial Feeds for The Young Infant.* Report on Health and Social Subjects, No.18. HMSO, London.

Individual Nutrients

2
Water

Water is quantitatively and qualitatively the single most important nutrient. Its requirement is not primarily determined by metabolic rate but by insensible water loss, renal concentrating power and renal solute load. In the very low birth weight (VLBW) infant water requirements are extremely variable and depend upon gestational age, postnatal age and environmental conditions. If one can first agree on the volume of water required to maintain health under prevailing conditions within a clearly defined thermal environment one can then decide on what should go into the water, and in what proportions, to maintain growth and health.

NUTRITIONAL BACKGROUND

Factors affecting water requirements

In a growing VLBW infant water requirements are determined by the amount of water lost from the body by various routes (insensible water loss, faecal water, urine water), and to a lesser extent by the amount retained in newly synthesized tissue.

Water for growth

From 26 to 36 weeks of intrauterine life, water represents about 70–80% of the weight gain(1), but from metabolic balance studies in preterm infants(2–5) water may comprise only 50–70% of the weight gain, similar to the proportion of water retained by the full term neonate during the first 3 months of postnatal life(6). Thus, assuming a growth rate of 15 g/kg per day, the amount deposited for growth is about 10 ml/kg per day. This is a small volume in relation to total water requirements and is almost equal to the daily water produced by nutrient oxidation, which amounts to around 12 ml/100 kcal oxidized.

Water losses

Water requirement is mainly determined by the amount of water lost from the body, which may be *extrarenal* (i.e. losses through the skin and respiratory tract, referred to as insensible water loss, and fecal water loss) which cannot be regulated, and *renal* which is subject to regulation.

Extrarenal water losses

    Insensible water loss (IWL) is very variable: it decreases with increasing body weight(7,8), gestational age(7–11) and postnatal age(7,8). It is increased by a rise in body temperature(12), low relative humidity(10,13), high ambient temperature(8,14,15) and high body activity(12). In a single walled incubator set to maintain a thermoneutral environment(16) with a relative humidity of 50–80%, IWL is estimated at between 30 and 60 ml/kg per day(8,15,17) after the first 10 days of life. These values have been used in our calculations of minimum water requirement. However, all studies show that IWL is higher during the first 10 days of life, particularly in VLBW infants less than 30 weeks gestation at birth(7,10).

    Water losses in faeces are almost constant (except during diarrhoea) and are estimated at 5–10 ml/kg per day(18–20).

    Thus under normal circumstances, for an infant nursed in an incubator after the first 10 days of life, total extrarenal water loss can be estimated at between 35–70 ml/kg per day (Table 2.1).

Renal water losses

The urinary water volume is determined mainly by water intake, extrarenal water loss and, in some circumstances, by renal solute load. It is modulated by the renal capability to concentrate or to dilute urine, which matures with advancing post-conceptional age(21–24). Indeed VLBW infants cannot concentrate their urine much above 400–500 mosmol/kg H_2O even with maximum vasopressin secretion(25) and therefore it is important to consider the relationship between urine volume and renal solute load. In order to demonstrate this, we have calculated (see appendix) a theoretical maximum and minimum renal solute load of the diet(26) using our maximum and minimum recommended nutrient requirements, and from these data the obligatory urinary output has been computed for various urine concentrations (Fig. 2.1).

    In practice a mean urinary concentration value of 150 mosmol/l (a range of 100–200 mosmol/l) is usually found in VLBW infants fed human milk or full term formula(19,27) and allows the infants to respond to changing water balance. A theoretical solute load of 14 mosmol/kg per day (see appendix) can be used to calculate a renal water loss of around 90 ml/kg per day under which there will be no excessive renal stress (see Fig. 2.1).

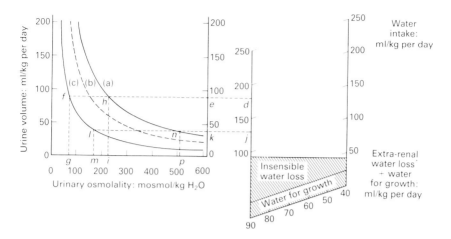

Fig. 2.1. The diagram on the left side describes the relationship between urinary osmolality and urine volume at different solute loads (see appendix): Maximum, average and minimum solute loads are indicated by lines (a), (b), (c). The lines joining the values of urine osmolality on the abscissa to lines (a), (b), and (c) indicate the urinary water which is necessary to dispose of any given solute load at the corresponding urinary osmolality.

The corresponding water intake which has to be provided depending on the extra renal water loss can be found by extrapolation to the diagram on the right side. Alternatively when water intake and extra water loss are known, it is possible to extrapolate the corresponding value of urinary volume and urinary osmolality for any given solute load.

For example, suppose a child has a water intake of 180 ml/kg per day and an extra renal water loss of 90 ml/kg per day (point *d*), the urine volume is 90 ml/kg per day (*e*). If the formula has the minimum solute load (*f*) the urine osmolality will be 72 mosmol/kg H_2O (*g*). If the formula has the maximum solute load (*h*) the urine osmolality will be 225 mosmol/kg H_2O (*i*).

If on the other hand the child has a lower water intake (130 ml/kg per day) but the extra renal water loss is still high at 90 ml/kg per day (*j*) the urine volume will be 40 ml/kg per day (*k*). If the formula has the minimum solute load (*l*) urinary osmolality will be 162 mosmol/kg H_2O (*m*). If the formula has the maximum solute load (*n*) the urinary osmolality will be 507 mosmol/kg H_2O (*p*).

(a) Maximum renal solute load curve (20.3 mosmol/kg per day)
(b) Average renal solute load curve (13.4 mosmol/kg per day)
(c) Minimum renal solute load curve (6.5 mosmol/kg per day) (see Appendix)

*Assuming that gastrointestinal water loss equals endogenous water production, extrarenal water loss is equivalent to insensible water loss (see Table 2.1).

Theoretical lower and upper limits of water intake

From the above data, the theoretical minimal water requirement can be calculated to be 130–160 ml/kg per day for a growing preterm infant receiving 130 kcal/kg per day (Table 2.1).

The theoretical upper limit on water intake is the renal capacity to eliminate water, which depends on renal glomerula filtration and renal dilution capacity. Glomerular filtration is low in premature infants(21) but their renal

Table 2.1.   Minimal water requirements (ml/kg per day) for
growing premature infants nursed in an incubator (thermoneutral
environment with a relative humidity 50–80%)[a].

Extra renal water loss:		
Insensible water loss (IWL)	30–60	
Gastro-intestinal water loss	5–10	
Renal water loss	90	
TOTAL WATER LOSS		125–160
Water for growth	10	
TOTAL REQUIREMENT		135–170
Water from endogenous sources	5–10	
MINIMAL WATER REQUIREMENT[b]		130–160

[a]Energy expenditure is assumed to be 40–80 kcal/kg per day, urine
    osmolality 150 mosmol/kg H_2O and renal solute load
    14 mosmol/kg per day

[b]If under phototherapy, add 15–30 ml to IWL.
    If infant nursed under radiant heater add 15–30 ml to IWL.

dilution capacity is good and they are able to excrete urine with an osmolality as
low as 60 mosmol/kg H_2O(24,28). Though some infants have received from
220 to 300 ml of milk per kg/d(23,29–31) without any problems, it has been
suggested that high fluid intakes during the first week of life may be associated
with a higher incidence of symptomatic patent ductus arteriosus(32,33),
necrotizing enterocolitis(33) and pulmonary oedema(34); this has not been
confirmed in a recent prospective study(35) but in this study fluid intake was
below 150 ml/kg per day during the first two weeks of life when these problems
are most likely to occur.

Special clinical conditions affecting water requirements

Heatshield, radiant heater

In a single walled incubator and in a comparable thermal environment, IWL
can be reduced by about 30% if a heatshield is placed over the infant(8,17,36).
If an infant is nursed under a radiant heater, increases in IWL of between 40
and 190% have been reported(36,37–39) but this rise can be partly reduced by
a heatshield(36,37,40).

Phototherapy

During phototherapy an increase in IWL of 40–50%(38,41) or even higher(39) has been reported. A VLBW infant nursed under a radiant heater and on phototherapy may have IWL twice as high as he would have if nursed within an incubator(38,39). Phototherapy is used mainly during the first 10 days of life when IWL is at its highest(7,8), so it is common practice to increase water intake by 20–40 ml/kg per day(18,33).

Heart failure

Some infants in heart failure may require fluid restriction; a total fluid intake (intravenous and oral) as low as 122 ± 14 ml/kg per day has been given to preterm infants throughout the first month of life(33) but a certain number of them became dehydrated. If careful attention is taken to minimize extrarenal water loss, it is likely that, after the first two weeks of life, water intake can be dropped to its minimum, i.e. 130 ml/kg per day (Table 2.1), without exceeding renal concentrating ability. However, this may result in inadequate food intake and poor growth if the nutrient density of the diet is too low.

REQUIREMENTS AND ADVISABLE INTAKE

The dry weight of human milk or formula is approximately 13% of the total by weight; therefore 100 ml of feed provides approximately 87 ml of water. However, water is also provided by oxidation of nutrients in the body in the amount of 12 ml/100 kcal. Therefore in practice it is usual to assume that the water intake is equivalent to the volume of feed.

Recommendations of other bodies

150 to 200 ml/kg per day is the usual amount of milk recommended during oral alimentation(42–44). This is in agreement with the average volume of milk given in most of the nutritional balances studies performed on orally fed VLBW infants(2–5,19,45) where adequate growth was documented without metabolic imbalance.

Recommendations

1 Adequate control of IWL is essential.
2 150 ml/kg per day of feed can be considered as the lower limit in normal circumstances; it meets our suggested mean energy intake of 130 kcal/kg per day when using a formula with our highest recommended energy density of 85 kcal/dl.

3 200 ml/kg of feed can be considered as an upper limit of volume intake; it provides 130 kcal/kg per day with a formula with our lowest recommended energy density of 65 kcal/kg per day.

4 In some clinical conditions lower or higher water intake may be necessary:

(a) Higher intake may be required in infants who have high insensible water losses (nursed under radiant warmers, phototherapy), especially during the first weeks of life.

(b) In infants with high energy requirements (small for gestational age (SGA) infants for instance) and fed on low energy density formula or human milk, higher intakes are sometimes needed in order to promote adequate growth.

(c) Lower intakes may sometimes be necessary (for instance in heart failure). An intake of 130 ml/kg per day at our recommended maximum energy density of 85 kcal/dl would provide 110 kcal/kg per day, which is our minimum recommended energy intake.

GUIDELINES

1 An intake of 180 ml/kg per day (range 150–200 ml) of human milk or formula meets the water requirements of VLBW infants under normal circumstances.

2 Higher intakes are not usually necessary.

3 Lower intakes may be necessary in certain clinical conditions. Fluid intake below 130 ml/kg per day should not be given without careful attention to IWL, thermoregulation and to the renal solute load, and may not meet the energy requirement.

APPENDIX

Calculations of the renal solute load (RSL) of a formula using the simple method of Ziegler & Fomon(46) are based on a growing full term infant of 4–7 kg fed cow's milk, and some of the assumption in their calculations are not appropriate for growing preterm infants. Therefore we have calculated the RSL of formula assuming an average nitrogen retention of 320 mg/kg.d, a sodium retention of 1 mmol/kg.d and a potassium retention of 0.7 mmol/kg.d; these values are based on estimates of intrauterine growth(1). Thus RSL was calculated from the following equation(26):

Total urine solute	=	urine urea	+	2 (Urinary Na	+	Urinary K)
(mosmol/kg per day)		(mmol/kg per day)		(mmol/kg per day)		(mmol/kg per day)

We made the calculations of the maximum and minimum RSL of a theoretical formula using our maximum and minimum recommended intake of protein, sodium and potassium, assuming that the absorption rate is 90%, and that any solute not retained for growth is excreted in the urine:

Minimum renal solute load: 6.5 mosmol/kg per day. We assume the lowest recommended volume intake in normal circumstances (150 ml/kg per day) of a formula with the lowest recommended potassium content (1.5 mmol/dl) providing the minimum recommended intake of sodium (1.3 mmol/kg) and of protein (2.9 g/kg) per day.

Maximum renal solute load: 20.3 mosmol/kg per day. We assume the highest recommended volume intake (200 ml/kg per day) of a formula with the highest recommended sodium and potassium content (1.5 and 2.5 mmol/dl, respectively), and which would provide 4 g/kg per day of protein (maximum recommended intake).

The guidelines mention that sodium supplements of up to 4 mmol per kg/d may be necessary. This could theoretically increase the renal solute load to 28 mosmol/kg per day and the urine concentration accordingly. However, if the babies retain any of this extra sodium it will not contribute to the renal osmolar load.

Average renal solute load: 13.4 mosmol/kg per day We assume a volume intake of 175 ml/kg of a formula with a protein content of 2 g/dl (i.e. providing 3.5 g/kg per day of protein) and a Na and K content of 1.2 and 2 mmol/dl respectively.

RSL calculation: average renal solute load (kg/d)

	Nitrogen (Prot. $\times$ 6.25) (mg)	Na (mmol)	K (mmol)
Intake	560	2.1	3.5
Absorbed	504	1.9	3.2
Retained	320	1.0	0.7
Lost in urine	184	0.9	2.5
Urinary solute load (mosmol)	6.6*	0.9	2.5

TOTAL RSL: 6.6 + 2 (0.9 + 2.5) = 13.4 mmol/kg per day

*assuming all nitrogen is derived from urea.

REFERENCES

1. Ziegler E.E., O'Donnell A., Nelson S.E. & Fomon S.J. (1976). Body composition of the reference fetus. *Growth* **40**, 329–41.
2. Whyte R.K., Haslam R., Vlainic C., Shannon S., Samulski K., Campbell D., Bayley H.S. &

Sinclair J.C. (1983). Energy balance and nitrogen balance in growing low birth weight infants fed human milk or formula. *Pediatr. Res.* **17**, 891–8.

3. Reichman B., Chessex P., Putet G., Verellen G., Smith J.M., Heim T. & Swyer P. (1981). Diet, fat accretion and growth in premature infants. *N. Engl. J. Med.* **305**, 1495–1500.

4. Reichman B., Chessex P., Verrellen G., Putet G., Smith J.M., Heim T. & Swyer P. (1983). Dietary composition and macronutrient storage in preterm infants. *Pediatrics* **72**, 322–8.

5. Putet G., Senterre J., Rigo J. & Salle B. (1984). Nutrient balance, energy utilization and composition of weight gain in very low birth weight infants fed pooled human milk or a preterm formula. *J. Pediatr.* **105**, 79–85.

6. Fomon S.J. (1967). Body composition of the male reference infant during the first year of life. *Pediatrics* **40**, 863–70.

7. Rutter N. & Hull D. (1979). Water loss from the skin of term and preterm babies. *Arch Dis. Child.* **54**, 858–68.

8. Fanaroff A.A., Wald M., Gruber H.S. & Klauss M.H. (1972). Insensible water loss in low birth weight infants. *Pediatrics* **49**, 236–45.

9. Hammarlund K. & Sedin G. (1979). Transepidermal water loss in newborn infants: III relation to gestational age. *Acta Paediatr. Scand.* **68**, 795–801.

10. Hammarlund K. & Sedin G. (1982). Transepidermal water loss in newborn infants. VI. Heat exchange with the environment in relationship to gestational age. *Acta Paediatr. Scand.* **71**, 191–6.

11. Wilson D.R. & Maibach H.I. (1980). Transepidermal water loss *in vivo*. Premature and term infants. *Biol. Neonate* **37**, 180–5.

12. Hammarlund K., Nilsson G.E., Öberg P.A. & Sedin G. (1979). Transepidermal water loss in newborn infants. II: relation to activity and body température. *Acta Paediatr. Scand.* **68**, 371–6.

13. Hammarlund K., Nilsson G.E., Oberg P.A. & Sedin G. (1977). Transepidermal water loss in newborn infants. I. relation to ambient temperature and site of measurement and estimation of total transepidermal water loss. *Acta Paediatr. Scand.* **66**, 553–62.

14. Harpin V.A. & Rutter N. (1982). Sweating in preterm babies. *J. Pediatr.* **100**, 614–19.

15. Bell E.F., Gray J.C., Weinstein M.R. & Oh W. (1980). The effects of thermal environment on heat balance and insensible water loss in low-birth-weight infants. *J. Pediatr.* **96**, 452–9.

16. Hey E.N. & Katz G. (1970). The optimum thermal environment for naked babies. *Arch. Dis. Child.* **45**, 328.

17. Yeh T.F., Lilien L.D., Matwynshyn J., Srinivasan G. & Pildes R.S. (1980). Oxygen consumption and insensible water loss in premature infants in single versus double walled incubators. *J. Pediatr.* **97**, 967–71.

18. Friiss Hansen B. (1983). Water distribution in the fetus and newborn infant. *Acta Paediatr. Scand.* (Suppl.) **305**, 7–11.

19. Senterre J. (1976). *Alimentation Optimale du Prématuré*. Vaillant Carmanne, Liège.

20. Oh W. & Karecki H. (1972). Phototherapy and insensible water loss in the newborn infant. *Am. J. Dis. Child.* **124**, 230–2.

21. Arant B.S. (1978). Developmental patterns of renal functional maturation compared in the human neonate. *J. Pediatr.* **92**, 705–12.

22. Ross B., Cowett R. & Oh W. (1977). Renal function of low birth weight infants during the first two months of life. *Pediatr. Res.* **11**, 1162–4.

23. Sulyok E., Varga F., Györy E., Jobst K. & Csaba I.F. (1979). Post-natal development of renal sodium handling in premature infants. *J. Pediatr.* **95**, 787–92.

24. Aperia A., Broberger O., Herin P., Thodenius K. & Zetterstrom R. (1983). Post-natal control of water and electrolyte homeostasis in preterm and full term infants. *Acta Paediatr. Scand.* (Suppl.) **305**, 61–5.

25. Rees L., Brook C.G.D., Shaw J.C.L. & Forsling M.L. (1984). Causes of hyponatremia in the first week of life in preterm infants. I – arginine vasopressin secretion. *Arch. Dis. Child.* **59**, 414–22.

26. Shaw J.C.L., Jones A. & Gunther M. (1973). Mineral content of brands of milk for infant feeding. *Brit. Med. J.* 2, 12–15.
27. Shenai J.P., Reynolds J.W. & Balson S.G. (1980). Nutritional balance studies in very low birth weight infants: Enhanced nutrient retention rates by an experimental formula. *Pediatrics* 66, 233–8.
28. Rodriguez-Soriano J., Vallo A., Oliveros R. & Castillo E. (1983). Renal handling of sodium in premature and full-term neonates: a study using clearance methods during water diuresis. *Pediatr. Res.* 17, 1013–16.
29. Brooke O.G., Alvear J. & Arnold M. (1979). Energy retention, energy expenditure and growth in healthy immature infants. *Pediatr. Res.* 13, 215–20.
30. Brooke O.G., Wood C. & Barley J. (1982). Energy balance, nitrogen intake and growth in preterm infants fed expressed breast milk, a premature infant formula and two low solute adapted formulae. *Arch. Dis. Child.* 12, 898–904.
31. Lewis M.A. & Smith B.A.M. (1984). High volume milk feeds for preterm infants. *Arch. Dis. Child.* 59, 779–81.
32. Stevenson J.G. (1977). Fluid administration in the association of patent ductus arteriosus complicating respiratory distress syndrome. *J. Pediatr.* 90, 257–61.
33. Bell E.F., Warburton D., Stonestreet B.S. & Oh W. (1980). Effects of fluid administration on the development of symptomatic patent ductus arteriosus and congestive heart failure in premature infant. *N. Engl. J. Med.* 302, 598–604.
34. Brown E.R., Stark A., Sosenko I., Lawson E.E. & Avery M.E. (1978). Broncho pulmonary dysplasia: possible relationship to pulmonary edema. *J. Pediatr.* 92, 982–4.
35. Lorenz J.M., Kleinman L.I., Kotagal U.R. & Reller M.D. (1982). Water balance in very low-birth-weight infants: Relationship to water and sodium intake and effect on outcome. *J. Pediatr.* 101, 423–32.
36. Bell E.F., Weinstein M.R. & Oh W. (1980). Heat balance in premature infants: comparative effects of convectively heated incubator and radiant warmer, with and without plastic heat shield. *J. Pediatr.* 96, 460–5.
37. Yeh T.F., Amma P., Lilien L.D., Baccaro M.M., Matwynshyn J., Pyati S. & Pildes R.S. (1979). Reduction of insensible water loss in premature infants under the radiant warmer. *J. Pediatr.* 94, 651–3.
38. Bell E.F., Neidich G.A., Cashore W.J. & Oh W. (1979). Combined effect of radiant warmer and phototherapy on insensible water loss in low-birth-weight infants. *J. Pediatr.* 94, 810–13.
39. Wu Pyk & Hodgman J.E. (1974). Insensible water loss in Preterm infants: changes in postnatal development and non-ionizing radiant energy. *Pediatrics* 54, 704–12.
40. Baumgart S., Engle N., Fox W. & Polin R.A. (1981). Effect of heat shielding on convective and evaporative heat losses and on radiant heat transfer in the premature infant. *J. Pediatr.* 99, 948–56.
41. Engle W.D., Baumgart S., Schwartz J.G., Fox W.W. & Polin R.A. (1981). Insensible water loss in the critically ill neonate: combined effect of Radiant-Warmer power and Phototherapy. *Am. J. Dis. Child.* 135, 516–20.
42. American Academy of Pediatrics – Committee on Nutrition (1977). Nutritional needs of low-birth-weight infants. *Pediatrics* 60, 519–30.
43. Canadian Pediatric Society – Nutrition Committee (1981). Feeding the low-birth-weight infant. *Can. Med. Assoc. J.* 124, 1301–10.
44. American Academy of Pediatrics – Committee on Nutrition (1985). Nutritional needs of low-birth weight infants. *Pediatrics* 75, 976–85.
45. Gross S.J. (1983). Growth and biochemical response of preterm infants fed human milk or modified infant formula. *N. Engl. J. Med.* 308, 237–41.
46. Ziegler E.E. & Fomon S. (1971). Fluid intake, renal solute load and water balance in infancy. *J. Pediatr.* 78, 561–8.

3
Energy

NUTRITIONAL BACKGROUND

Evaluation of the energy (E) requirement of the growing orally-fed preterm infant can be based on the study of the energy balance equation:

$$E \text{ intake} = E \text{ stored} + E \text{ expended} + E \text{ excreted}$$

where:

   E intake is the E provided by the food.

   E stored is the E laid down as fat and protein and other components in newly formed tissue.

   E expended comprises the energy used for resting metabolism, thermo-regulation, activity and for the synthesis of new tissue.

   E excreted occurs mainly in the faeces (and to a small extent in the urine).

   E cost of growth includes E utilized for synthesis of new tissues and E stored in these new tissues.

   E for maintenance is the minimal E expenditure within a thermoneutral environment, when no growth occurs.

Most of the information available about each part of this equation has been derived from short-term measurements and it is difficult to assess the impact of the results quantitatively over longer periods. However, a precise estimation of each term of the E balance equation should lead to a reasonable overall evaluation of the E requirements.

Energy stored during growth

Several studies (1–5) have examined the tissue composition of the fetus at different gestational ages. From calculations of fat and protein accretion during fetal growth, a value of 20 to 30 kcal/kg may be estimated to be stored every day in new tissues as body weight increases from 1 kg to 3.5 kg. These calculated values vary slightly within the indicated range according to gestational age and assume a mean daily weight gain of 15 g/kg.

The value of such calculations in estimating the E requirements for extrauterine growth needs to be examined. The estimation of E stored is based on the assumption (a) that adequate growth of the preterm newborn should imitate intrauterine quantitatively, an assumption which has already been reviewed in Chapter 1; and (b) that for the same weight gain, the quality of this gain (estimated as the amount of fat and protein deposited per g of weight gain) is identical *in utero* and during extrauterine life in the orally-fed preterm infant. However, a comparison of the composition of tissue deposited by the fetus(1) and the composition of weight gained by the full term infant during the first two months of extrauterine life(6) shows quite a different pattern in the two situations, with more fat and less water being deposited during extrauterine life. Furthermore, results from balance studies in the growing, formula-fed, preterm infant on high energy intakes(7–11) seem to show the same trends with a greater amount of fat being deposited during extrauterine growth. Thus the estimation of daily stored energy, based on existing data of fetal composition, can only be a guide, as it has not yet been shown to be possible or necessary to mimic intrauterine growth qualitatively during extrauterine life.

Energy expended

This includes energy for *resting* metabolism, *muscular activity*, *thermoregulation* and E expended for *synthesis* of new tissue.

Resting energy expenditure

In older infants or in adults, basal metabolic rate (BMR) is the usual reference for comparison of metabolic rates and is properly measured after overnight fasting (12–18 hours). As premature infants should not be fasted for long periods of time, resting metabolic rate (RMR) is the usual comparative measurement. In this particular case, RMR differs from BMR in that it includes a part of energy used for growth(12), even when measured just prior to the next feed, because the interval between feeds is short. In consequence, RMR is in part dependent on the energy intake. This may explain differences in results reported in the literature, where RMR estimations (measured either by indirect or direct calorimetry) vary from 45 to 60 kcal/kg per day (12–17), lower values being reported(18,19) especially during the first 2 weeks of life(18). It is generally agreed that RMR rises during the first weeks of life(12,13,16,17,20,21) probably due to increasing E intake(22), and is higher in SGA than in AGA infants(16).

Intermittent activity

Most of the variations in energy expended for spontaneous activity is accounted for by the thermal environment, gestational age and postnatal age (because the more immature the neonate the more time he spends asleep and because for a given activity more energy seems to be expended with increased postnatal age (14,15)). Over short periods, maximum activity levels have been shown to increase RMR two to three times(23) but measurements of the energy cost over 24 hours are more difficult to achieve. By measuring metabolic rate during different activity levels and by documenting the proportion of time spent in these states, Brooke estimated energy cost of activity in LBW infants between 13 to 19 kcal/kg per day(15). Another way of estimating it is to measure the global E expended over prolonged periods. If care is taken to assure a thermoneutral environment and to take into account the energy cost of growth (or to perform the study during a period of no growth) it can be assumed that the only E expended will be for maintenance (i.e., RMR and activity, see Table 3.1). With measurements of this kind, activity cost has been estimated at 4.3 kcal/kg per day by Reichman(13) and 6 kcal/kg per day by Mestyan(18). Variations therefore exist between different estimations(24,25) and an activity cost of 10 kcal/kg per day(24) seems acceptable since it is likely that during some of the studies cited(13,18) handling of the infants was decreased by comparison with normal nursing conditions, especially in the older ones.

Table 3.1. Estimation of energy requirement of the LBW infant

	Range kcal/kg per day	Average estimation kcal/kg per day	
E EXPENDED			
Resting metabolic rate	45–60	52.5	*E* for
Activity	5–10	7.5	maintenance
Thermoregulation	5–10	7.5	
Synthesis	10–25	17.5	*E* cost of
E STORED*	20–30	25.0	growth
E EXCRETED	10–30	20.0	
E INTAKE	95–165**	130.0	

*Calculated for an average daily weight gain of 15g/kg.d
**See discussion, lower limit revised to 110 kcal/kg.d

Thermoregulation

Heat is lost by convection, radiation, evaporation and conduction. Under normal circumstances the major routes of heat loss are radiation and convection, but occasionally evaporation may become important, for example if an infant is ventilated with inadequate humidity. Most of the data on the influence of cold exposure on E expenditure have been collected over short periods of time with acute exposure to cold (26–28) and have been recently reviewed in a monograph(29). Two- to threefold increases in metabolic rate have been described in these situations. Studies on the effect of minimal but more chronic cold stress are rare. In a study by Glass(30) caloric expenditure was 7 to 8 kcal/kg per day greater in infants nursed just below the thermoneutral range than in those who were adequately warmed. Cold stress can be minimized in an incubator with careful adherence to standard methods for maintaining a thermoneutral environment(31). However, it has been shown(32) that nurses' estimation of a good thermal environment might be erroneous and that they elect to keep the infants in a slightly cool environment with a rise of their O_2 consumption rate. Furthermore, thermal losses might increase when a sick premature infant is handled frequently, or when an older growing premature infant is bathed and nursed. Therefore the value of 10 kcal/kg per day(24,25,33) is likely to cover requirements of incidental cold stress and a range of 5–10 kcal/kg per day is an acceptable estimation for E lost in thermoregulation.

Energy for synthesis

E cost of growth includes (see Table 3.1) E utilized for synthesis of new tissues and E stored in these new tissues, values for the latter having been already derived. Estimation of the E required for synthesis is rather difficult as results from the literature are controversial. It will vary with the composition of new tissue deposited. In one review(14) data for E for synthesis vary from 0.26 to 1.1 kcal per gram of weight gain(14,34). In a re-evaluation of the E requirement for growth and using Atkinson's metabolic price system, Hommes(35) estimated that 2.1% of the total daily energy intake (i.e. 0.3 kcal/g of weight gain) is used to cover these needs for synthetic processes in his male reference term newborn. In recent studies using techniques of energy balance and indirect calorimetry in LBW infants, requirements for synthesis have been estimated at 0.55 (19), 0.67 (13) and 1.7 (15) kcal per g weight gain. Assuming an average weight gain of 15 g/kg per day the E cost for synthesis would vary from around 10 (13,19) to 25 (15) kcal/kg per day. Using Kielanowski's constants (36), Sinclair (12) estimated the E cost for synthesis in LBW infants at 11 kcal/kg per day. Obviously more studies are needed for a better evaluation of E required for synthesis. For the moment we estimate 10 to 25 kcal/kg per day to be an acceptable range of E expended for synthesis.

Energy excreted

Energy excretion occurs mainly in the faeces due to fat and nitrogen losses, the major factor being the well known fat malabsorption of the LBW infant (see Chapter 5). When the energy intake is increased there is a decrease in the proportion of E absorbed (37) and although net energy retention rises, faecal E losses also increase. From the results of various E balance studies (7–11,13,38), E excretion varies from 10 kcal/kg per day (13,15) to as much as 70 kcal/kg per day (15). However, an average retention of 80 to 90% of the E intake may be expected by two to three weeks of age. Thus excretory losses may vary from 10 to 30 kcal/kg per day.

ENERGY IN AVAILABLE FOOD

The energy density of human milk has an average value of 65–70 kcal/dl. Although there have been reports that the E density of preterm milk is greater than term milk (39,40), most of the data seem to indicate that there is little difference in the energy content (41–44), but that variability is greater (44). Fat digestion has been said to be better with fresh human milk than with formula (45) (see Chapter 5), increasing the net E retention. Pooled human milk, especially when heat-treated, might lose some of these nutritional advantages, as recently underlined (46,47). Ideally, the E content of human milk should be monitored because large variations have been shown, particularly with pooled human milk (48) and with preterm milk (48,49). It is also known that E may be lost as fat deposited on the syringe and delivery tubing during tube feeding (50).

Adapted formulas have an average E content of 70 kcal/dl. The optimal E density of formulas fed to preterm infants has yet to be determined, but under some circumstances it may be desirable to increase the density. Since the volume of milk given to meet the E requirement may be a problem because of small gastric capacity or fluid intolerance, more concentrated formulas (up to 90 kcal/dl) have been marketed. These formulas may have the disadvantage of causing a higher renal solute load and of having a higher osmolality than standard formulas. Formulas specially prepared for the preterm infant offer a fat composition aimed at minimizing faecal fat losses, often using medium chain triglycerides, thus raising the E retention without a higher solute load. However, complications have been described with high energy formulas, especially the occurrence of fat lactobezoars (51,52).

ESTIMATION OF ENERGY REQUIREMENT

An estimation of the range of energy requirements derived from the above data is summarized in Table 3.1. The mean value of 130 kcal/kg per day fits in well with previous estimates (24) and recommendations from other committees (25,33). Energy requirements of the human fetus (53) have been estimated at 90–100 kcal/kg per day. Since in this situation there is no need for thermoregulation and since there is less activity and no excretory losses, these values are in agreement with the above calculations. The only factors which can be modified in order to increase the E available for growth for a given E intake are E expended in thermoregulation and E excreted in stools. These factors are thus of considerable practical importance.

From the above estimations an intake of 130 kcal/kg per day should meet the E requirements of most LBW infants, allowing a growth rate similar to intrauterine. When careful attention is paid to thermoregulation and when good fat absorption is obtained, these requirements may theoretically drop below 100 kcal/kg per day, but badly absorbed milk, poor temperature regulation, increased activity and high level of handling will all increase these E requirements and must be considered when setting an optimum energy intake. Therefore a *lower* limit of 110 kcal/kg per day is suggested. From the available data, 165 kcal/kg per day should be considered as the *upper* limit of E intake because above this value energy may be inadequately utilized and may not necessarily result in faster and/or better growth (37), but indeed may cause abnormally high fat deposition (7,10,13).

GUIDELINES

An E intake of 120–130 kcal/kg per day may be achieved with a volume of 180–200 ml/kg per day of expressed breast milk (EBM), or adapted formula if the E density is 65–70 kcal/dl. This energy density is that normally found in breast milk, so it can be considered as the minimum E density required for feeding LBW infants, since they usually tolerate the necessary volume intake well.

It is more difficult to set an upper level for E density. Since in some circumstances the infant's caloric requirements have to be met with lower than the usual volume of intake, it may be desirable to give a higher energy density than that of breast milk. Thus to achieve an energy intake of 130 kcal/kg per day at a fluid intake of 150–200 ml/kg per day, the energy density needs to be 65–85 kcal per 100 ml. We see no reason to exceed this limit.

It has been suggested that E supplements could be useful in the clinical management of LBW infants(54). However, careful consideration should be given to the relationship between nitrogen E intake in this situation(55): an increase in the E intake could lead to a relative protein deprivation if the protein content of the supplemented milk is already low, and if the supplement is protein-free (see Chapter 4).

SUMMARY OF GUIDELINES

1   An intake 130 kcal/kg per day (range 110–165 kcal/kg per day) meets the requirements of the LBW infant under normal circumstances.

2   This mean E intake may be provided by breast milk or an adapted formula of a similar energy density (i.e. 65–70 kcal per dl) in a volume of 180–200 ml/kg per day. If a higher E density is required a concentration of 85 kcal/dl should not be exceeded.

REFERENCES

1. Ziegler E.E., O'Donnell A., Nelson S.E. & Fomon S.J. (1976). Body composition of the reference fetus. *Growth* **40**, 329–41.
2. Widdowson E.M. (1968). Growth and composition of the fetus and newborn. In: *Biology of Gestation*. Vol. 2. (Ed. N.S. Assali) 1–49. Academic Press, New York.
3. Widdowson E.M. (1980). *Importance of Nutrient in Development with Special Reference to Feeding the Low Birth Weight Infant*. Proceedings of Ross Clinical Research Conference. Meeting nutritional goals for low birth weight infants. Tarpon Springs, Florida 1980.
4. Southgate D.A.T. & Hey E.N. (1976). In: *Biology of Human Fetal Growth*. (Eds D.F. Roberts & A.M. Thomson). Taylor & Francis, London.
5. Widdowson E.M. (1974). Changes in body proportions and composition during growth. In: *Scientific Foundations of Paediatrics* (Eds J.A. Davis & J. Dobbing) p. 153. Heinemann, London.
6. Fomon S.J. (1967). Body composition of the male reference infant during the first year of life. *Pediatrics* **40**, 863–70.
7. Reichman B., Chessex P., Putet G., Verellen G., Smith J., Heim T. & Swyer P.R. (1981). Diet, Fat accretion and growth in premature infants. *N. Eng. J. Med.* **305**, 1495–500.
8. Heim T., Verellen G., Chessex P., Putet G., Reichman B., Swyer P.R. & Smith J. (1983). Substrate utilization in the growing very low birth weight formula fed infant. In: *Intensive Care of the Newborn*, IV. pp. 169–81. Masson, New York.
9. Whyte R.K., Haslam R., Vlainic C., Shannon S., Samulski K., Campbell D., Bayley H.S. & Sinclair J.C. (1983). Energy balance and nitrogen balance in growing low birth weight infants fed human milk or formula. *Pediatr. Res.* **17**, 891–8.
10. Putet G., Senterre J., Rigo J. & Salle B. (1984). Nutrient balance, energy utilization and composition of weight gain in very-low-birth-weight infants fed pooled human milk or a preterm formula. *J. Pediatr.* **105**, 79–85.
11. Reichman B., Chessex P., Verellen G., Putet G., Smith J.M., Heim T. & Swyer P.R. (1983). Dietary composition and macronutrient storage in preterm infants. *Pediatrics* **72**, 322–8.
12. Sinclair J.C. (1978). Energy balance of the newborn. In: *Temperature Regulation and Energy Metabolism in the Newborn*. (Ed. J.C. Sinclair). pp. 187–204. Grune & Stratton, New York.
13. Reichman B.L., Chessex P.C., Putet G., Verellen G.J.E., Smith J.M., Heim T. & Swyer P.R. (1982). Partition of energy metabolism and energy cost of growth in the very low birth weight infant. *Pediatrics* **69**, 446–51.

14. Sauer P.J.J., Danee H.J., Pearse R.G. & Visser H.K.A. (1981). Energy requirements for growth in the neonate. In: *Metabolic Adaptation to Extrauterine Life*, (Ed. R. de Meyer) pp. 191–207. Martinus Nijhoff, The Hague.

15. Brooke O.G., Alvear J. & Arnold M. (1979). Energy retention, energy expenditure and growth in healthy immature infants. *Pediatr. Res.* **13**, 215–20.

16. Hill J.R. & Robinson D.C. (1968). Oxygen consumption in normally grown, small for date and large for date newborn infants. *J. Physiol.* **199**, 685–703.

17. Scopes J.W. & Ahmed I. (1966). Minimal rates of oxygen consumption in sick and premature newborn infants. *Arch. Dis. Child.* **4**, 407–16.

18. Mestyán J., Jarai I. & Fekete M. (1968). The total energy expenditure and its components in premature infants maintained under different nursing and environmental conditions. *Pediatr. Res.* **2**, 161–71.

19. Gudinchet F., Schutz Y., Micheli J.L., Stettler E. & Jecquier E. (1982). Metabolic cost of growth in the very low birth weight infants. *Pediatr. Res.* **16**, 1025–30.

20. Hill J.R. & Rahimtulla K.A. (1965). Heat balance and the metabolic rate of newborn babies in relation to environmental temperature and the effect of age and weight on basal metabolic rate. *J. Physiol.* **180**, 239–65.

21. Mestyán J. (1978). Energy metabolism and substrate utilization in the newborn. In: *Temperature Regulation and Energy Metabolism in the Newborn*. (Ed. J.C. Sinclair) 39–74. Grune & Stratton, New York.

22. Bhakoo O.N. & Scopes J.W. (1974). Minimal rates of oxygen consumption in small for date babies during the first week of life. *Arch. Dis. Child.* **49**, 583–5.

23. Rubecz I. & Mestyán J. (1975). Activity, energy metabolism and postnatal relationship in low birth weight infants. *Acta Paediatr. Acad. Sci. Hung.* **16**, 351–62.

24. Sinclair J.C., Driscoll J.M., Heird W.C. & Winters R.W. (1970). Supportive management of the sick neonate: parenteral calories, water electrolytes. *Pediatr. Clin. North Am.* **17**, 863.

25. American Academy of Pediatrics: Committee on Nutrition (1985). Nutritional needs of low birth weight infants. *Pediatrics* **75**, 976–86.

26. Scopes J.W. (1966). Metabolic rate and temperature control in the human baby. *Br. Med. Bull.* **22**, 88–91.

27. Brück K., Parmelee A.H. & Brück M. (1962). Neutral temperature range and range of thermal comfort in premature. *Biol. Neonate* **4**, 32–51.

28. Brück K. (1961). Temperature regulation in the newborn infant. *Biol. Neonate* **3**, 65–119.

29. Sinclair J.C., ed. (1978). *Temperature Regulation and Energy Metabolism in the Newborn*. Grune & Stratton, New York.

30. Glass L., Silverman W.A. & Sinclair J.C. (1968). Effect of the thermal environment on cold resistance and growth of the small infants after the first week of life. *Pediatrics* **41**, 1033–46.

31. Hey E.N. (1971). The care of babies in incubators. In: *Recent Advances in Pediatrics*, 4th Edn. (Eds. D. Gairdner & D. Hull) p. 171. Churchill Livingstone, London.

32. Smales O.R.C. (1978). Simple method for measuring oxygen consumption in babies. *Arch. Dis. Child.* **53**, 53–7.

33. Canadian Paediatric Society: Nutrition Committee (1981). Feeding the Low Birth Weight Infant. *Can. Med. Assoc. J* **124**, 1301–11.

34. Spady D.W., Payne P.R., Picou D. & Waterlow J.C. (1976). Energy balance during recovery from malnutrition. *Am. J. Clin. Nutr.* **29**, 1073–88.

35. Hommes F.A. (1980). The energy requirement for growth – a reevaluation. *Nutr. Metab.* **24**, 110–13.

36. Kielanowski J. (1965). Energy metabolism. In: *Proceedings of the Symposium on Energy Metabolism, Troon*. (Ed. K.L. Baxter). pp. 13–20. Academic Press, London.

37. Brooke O.G. (1980). Energy balance and metabolic rate in preterm infants fed with standard and high energy formulas. *Br. J. Nutr.* **44**, 13–23.

38. Brooke O.G., Wood C. & Barley J. (1982). Energy balance, nitrogen balance and growth in

preterm infants fed expressed breast milk a premature infant formula and two low solute adapted formulae. *Arch. Dis. Child.* 57, 898–904.

39. Guerrini P., Bosi G., Chierici R. & Fabbri A. (1981). Human milk: relationship of fat content with gestational age. *Early Hum. Dev.* 5, 187–94.

40. Anderson G.H., Atkinson S.A. & Bryan M.M. (1981). Energy and macronutrient content of human milk during early lactation from mothers giving birth prematurely and at term. *Am. J. Clin. Nutr.* 34, 258–65.

41. Lemons J.A., Moye L., Hall D. & Simmons M. (1982). Differences in the composition of preterm and term human milk during early lactation. *Pediatr. Res.* 16, 113–17.

42. Anderson D.M., Williams F.H., Merkatz R.B., Shulman P.K., Kerr D. & Pittard W.B. (1983). Length of gestation and nutritional composition of human milk. *Am. J. Clin. Nutr.* 37, 810–14.

43. Gross S.J., David R.J., Bauman L. & Tomarelli R.M. (1980). Nutritional composition of milk produced by mothers delivering preterm. *J. Pediatr.* 96, 641–4.

44. Hibberd C., Brooke O.G., Carter N.D. & Wood C. (1981). A comparison of protein concentration and energy in breast milk from preterm and term mothers. *J. Hum. Nutr.* 35, 189–98.

45. Alemi B., Hamosh M., Scanlon J.W., Salzman-Mann C. & Hamosh P. (1981). Fat digestion in very low birth weight infants: effect of addition of human milk to low birth weight formula. *Pediatrics* 68, 484–9.

46. Atkinson S.A., Bryan H. & Anderson G.H. (1981). Human milk feeding in premature infants: protein, fat and carbohydrate balances in the first two weeks of life. *J. Pediatr.* 99, 617–24.

47. Williamson S., Finucarne E., Ellis H. & Gasmu H.R. (1978). Effect of heat treatment of human milk on absorption of nitrogen, fat, sodium, calcium and phosphorus by preterm infants. *Arch. Dis. Child.* 53, 555–63.

48. Carrol L., Conlan D. & Davis D.P. (1980). Fat content of bank human milk. *Arch. Dis. Child.* 55, 969.

49. Hibberd C.M., Brooke O.G., Carter N.D., Haug M. & Harzer G. (1982). Variation in the composition of breast milk during the first weeks of lactation: implication for the feeding of preterm infants. *Arch. Dis. Child.* 57, 658–62.

50. Brooke O.G. & Barley J. (1978). Loss of energy during continuous infusion of breast milk. *Arch. Dis. Child.* 53, 344–5.

51. Duritz G. & Oltorf C. (1979). Lactobezoar formation associated with high density caloric formula. *Pediatrics* 63, 647–50.

52. Errenberg A., Shaw R.D. & Yousef-Zadeh D. (1979). Lactobezoar in the low birth weight infant. *Pediatrics* 63, 642–6.

53. Sparks J.W., Girard J.R. & Battaglia F.C. (1980). An estimate of the caloric requirements of the human fetus. *Biol. Neonate* 38, 113–19.

54. Raffles A., Schiller G., Erhardt P. & Silverman M. (1983). Glucose polymer supplementation of feeds for very low birth weight infants. *Br. Med. J.* 286, 935–6.

55. Senterre J. (1976). *Alimentation Optimale du Prématuré.* (Ed. Vaillant Carmanne S.A.) Liège.

4

Protein

NUTRITIONAL BACKGROUND

There are four major considerations affecting the quantity and quality of protein to be given to a low birth weight (LBW) baby:
  (a) requirements for normal growth and body composition;
  (b) development of protein and amino acid metabolism;
  (c) energy intake and available energy for growth;
  (d) renal function.

Requirements for normal growth and body composition

A number of different techniques have been used to estimate the requirements in preterm infants, e.g. the classical factorial method (1), postnatal growth rates (2–10), nitrogen balance (12–21), serum amino acid levels (8, 11–12, 22–27), body composition (15,21,28), labelled amino acid turnover (15,29,30), fractional nitrogen excretion (17), and calorimetry (21,28). The interpretation of these studies in the small infant is very difficult, because the optimal rate at which preterm infants *ex utero* should accumulate protein is yet to be determined.

The classical factorial method suggests that the amount of protein in human milk and many formulas designed for normal babies is inadequate for LBW babies (1). The calculations assume that the *in utero* growth rate *ex utero* remains optimal and that the body composition of the developing fetus is adequately known. There is, however, some circumstantial biochemical evidence of protein undernutrition in LBW babies undergoing rapid catch up growth (11,31) and some balance (12,15–16,18) and growth studies (2–6,10) have shown that babies fed expressed human milk retain less nitrogen and gain weight less quickly than those receiving a cow's milk-based formula. Others, however, have found no differences in nitrogen retention and net protein gain in preterm infants fed human milk or a formula containing more protein than that of breast milk (30). But the question remains, does a possible difference in weight gain have any advantage? Are the differences in weight gain due to the differences in protein intake or other factors, e.g. a lower energy content and a lower mineral content of human milk compared with cow's milk-based formulas.

Development of protein and amino acid metabolism

It is not sufficient merely to estimate protein requirements on the basis of theoretical calculations from *in utero* accumulation rates or to administer large quantities of protein in order to attain intrauterine growth rates in the immediate extrauterine environment. The biochemical immaturity of the human preterm infant makes him nutritionally very vulnerable, and the margin between an adequate protein intake and possible adverse effects of protein undernutrition or overnutrition is small. There is an incomplete development of several amino acid metabolic pathways in the newborn infant especially in the small preterm infant (32). The relevance of vitamin intake to this problem is discussed in the section on vitamins. Thus many of the amino acids previously thought to be non-essential may be essntial, at least for the immature organism and must be supplied in the diet, e.g. cysteine (23), taurine (23,24–26) and glycine (15). Also amino acid catabolism is incomplete and a high protein intake may result in high plasma concentrations of amino acids, hydrogen ion and ammonia (9, 22, 23, 25, 33). It is not conclusively established that these metabolic changes are harmful; indeed similar values have been found in fetal blood obtained at fetoscopy (34) or from umbilical at birth (35). Neither can it be conclusively said that they are harmless (36,37).

Energy intake and available energy for growth

Not only do the level and adequacy of the protein intake influence the status and rate of whole body protein metabolism, but nitrogen balance and stable isotope studies have shown that absorbed energy is also a key factor in determining the amount and rate of protein synthesized in the rapidly growing infant (38). If energy intake is inadequate, administration of protein in quantities which exceed the needs for synthesis stress the infant's metabolic machinery for disposing excess; on the other hand, if the amount of energy available for growth is adequate, the same protein intake can produce a higher weight gain and apparent nitrogen retention without deleterious metabolic effects. In classical terms the outcome depends on which is the 'limiting nutrient', protein or energy. The protein:energy ratio in a diet therefore also needs consideration.

AVAILABLE FOODS

Human milk

The proteins of human milk have been reviewed recently (39–41). The protein content of human milk is about 1.2 g/dl (1.8 g per 100 kcal) when expressed as total nitrogen x6.25 and about 0.9 g/dl (1.3 g per 100 kcal) (9,41,42) when expressed as true protein. The non-protein nitrogen (NPN) fraction in human milk constitutes about 25% of the total nitrogen. Transitional human milk (6–10 days postpartum) contains 1.6 g/dl and colostrum (first 5 days postpartum) 2.3 g/dl (40). The milk of women delivering prematurely contains approximately 20% more nitrogen for the first 14 days of lactation than milk of mothers delivering at term (43–46) but not all studies show this (44,45). The whey proteins represent more than 70% of the total proteins in human milk, but less than 20% in cows milk (47,48). β-lacto-globulin is the main whey protein in cow's milk but is absent from human milk which is rich in α-lactalbumin, lactoferrin and immunoglobulins. The whey proteins used in some formulas are thus very different in composition from the whey proteins in human milk. Human milk from milk banks can be enriched with components of human milk such as fat or protein, etc (human milk engineering) but further careful clinical evaluation is needed (49–51) (see Chapter 16 on the use of breast milk p. 201).

Cow's milk based formula

Most commercial formulas used for feeding healthy term infants have an energy density of 67 kcal/dl, and a protein content of 1.5–2.0 g/dl thus containing 2.2–3.0 g protein per 100 kcal. The protein is often whey-predominant (whey/casein 60:40) but there are a number of 'unadapted' cow's milk based formulas available with a whey/casein ratio of 18:82.

Formulas specifically designed for LBW infants have a higher energy density, usually from 75 to 81 kcal per dl but also a somewhat higher protein content, from 1.8 to 2.4 g per dl, than the formulas generally used for term infants. These formulas thus contain about 2.2–3.2 g protein per 100 kcal.

REQUIREMENTS AND ADVISABLE INTAKES

Despite its limitations (see Nutritional Background, p. 37), the factorial method of assessment provides a means to estimate requirements. As discussed above it provides no information about whether the amount provided in the diet can be absorbed or utilized after absorption. Intakes of 4.0 g per kg (3.1 per 100 kcal) for growth from 800 to 1200 g, and 3.5 g per kg (2.7 per 100 kcal) for growth from 1200 to 1800 g have been suggested (1), but experimental evidence that they can be used is lacking. On the other hand there is evidence that protein intakes from adapted formula of 2.7–3.0 g per kg, or 2.0–2.5 g per 100 kcal, support postnatal growth and nitrogen accumulation rates in LBW infants without acidosis, elevated BUN values or amino-acid aberrations (11,13,16,52).

Breast milk

Even if the protein content of breast milk is accepted as 1.2 g/dl (i.e. total nitrogen x6.25) a protein intake of 3.0 g could be achieved with mature human milk only with intakes above 250 ml/kg per day. Although such high intakes have been recorded (53) they are not in common use. The minimum intake of 2.25 g/kg per day recommended by the American Academy of Pediatrics, Committee on Nutrition (54) could, however, be achieved by feeding about 185 ml/kg per day. Intakes of 185–200 ml per kg per day are common practice and there is evidence that moderately LBW babies (>1.5 kg) thrive and achieve intrauterine rate of weight gain without signs of metabolic stress on such intakes (7,8,52). Recent studies have also shown considerably better fat absorption, larger intraluminal total bile acid concentration and greater bile acid pool size in preterm infants fed human milk (partially mothers own fresh milk) compared with infants fed some formulas (55–57). Not everyone has found this, however, particularly if the breast milk has been heat-treated (58). It has been suggested that heat-treated human milk which inactivates the milk lipase (59) is not ideal for VLBW infants, since it results in poor fat absorption, a less desirable protein nutritional status and a slow body weight gain. Several reports suggest that very LBW babies (<1.5 kg) may benefit in terms of better weight gain and nitrogen accumulation rate from fresh preterm milk, presumably because of its somewhat higher protein content (60,61).

In early life when the 'protective factors' in human milk may be of great value, we consider it is reasonable to accept the low protein content of breast milk, even though it is theoretically suboptimal. For this reason it is acceptable to provide breast milk or, better, the mother's own preterm milk fed at 185 ml/kg per day or more, assuming that any deficiencies of growth or body composition will be repaired after this critical period for survival is over (33). If there is inadequate weight gain and there is reason to suspect relative protein deficiency (e.g. total protein content of milk less than 1.2 g per 100 ml) then either the milk may be supplemented with protein (see section on breast milk p. 9) or with formula (50, 51).

Formulas

Formulas specially designed for LBW babies require thorough study and evaluation before routine use is justified, but the following guidelines may be helpful.

Lower limit

There is documented experience of feeding LBW babies with formulas containing 1.5 g protein and 80 kcal per dl, i.e. 1.9 per 100 kcal at a protein intake of 2.25 g per kg per day and these babies grew as well as babies receiving breast milk (9). The energy intake in this study was 118 kcal per kg, i.e. somewhat below our suggested target energy intake of 130 kcal per kg. We do not know whether this protein would still be adequate with a higher energy and sodium intake. We therefore do not at present suggest the general use of such a low protein:energy ratio, even though it is similar to that in breast milk. Many LBW babies receiving 130 kcal per kg from full-term formulas thrive and have little evidence of metabolic protein overload (13,16,52). In view of this, and the estimate of protein requirements made from body composition studies, there seems little argument for designing a LBW formula which contains less protein or has a lower protein:energy ratio than that for term babies. At present we suggest this as a lower limit, i.e. 1.5 g protein per dl, 2.25 g per 100 kcal, which if fed at 130 kcal per kg would provide 2.9 g per kg.

Upper limit

A protein concentration of about 3.1 g per 100 kcal has been proposed on theoretical grounds(1). A number of formulas are available with a protein: energy ratio as high as this but detailed documented experience, particularly data on metabolic tolerance (e.g. plasma concentration of ammonia, amino acids, urea, hydrogen ion, urinary concentrations) is very limited. If fed at the maximum recommended energy intake of 150 kcal per kg this would give an intake of 4.6 g per kg; this is not recommended. Even at lower total energy intakes, however, this high protein:energy ratio of 3.1 g per 100 kcal may be associated with problems. One study found that an intake of 3.0 g/100 kcal compared with an intake of 2.3 g/100 kcal (fed at 117 kcal per kg, i.e. 2.5–3.2 g per kg) did not lead to faster growth but a quarter of the babies developed late metabolic acidosis (33). At present we consider that formulas containing more than 3.0 g of protein per 100 kcal, more than 2 g/dl, should be used with caution, particularly during the first weeks or so of life, until additional systematically recorded experience becomes available. Formulas with protein content greater than this, e.g. 3.8 g per 100 kcal (3 g, 78 kcal per dl fed at 150 ml per kg, i.e. 117 kcal and 4.5 g protein per kg day) are associated with high plasma concentrations of aromatic amino acid, ammonia and hydrogen ion, particularly if the protein is mainly casein (9,25). These high intakes are not recommended.

Protein quality

Whey-predominant formulas are associated with lower plasma aromatic amino acid concentration (11,25) and when fed at an intake of 3.0 g protein and 134 kcal per kg per day with greater nitrogen absorption and more rapid growth (13). At the present time all formulas intended for LBW infants are whey-predominant. However, this may change in the future when more clinical investigations on this question have been performed. A whey-predominant formula will ensure an intake of cysteine at least that of the breast-fed baby. However, the increased threonine intake is associated with increased plasma concentrations of threonine in babies receiving those formulas (22,62). Also demineralized whey is more sensitive to blockage of lysine (Maillard reaction) during sterilization (see Chapter 17).

LBW infants who receive dietary taurine (e.g. in breast milk or added to a formula) when compared to infants on a conventional taurine free formula, excrete taurine in the urine and have higher values for plasma taurine concentrations, intraluminal bile acid concentrations, and duodenal bile acid taurine:glycine ratios (23,26,56,57,63). Nevertheless, although these may be good arguments in favour of supplementing formulas intended for LBW infants with taurine, until more definite *clinical* evidence in human infants for a clear benefit of taurine supplementation is found, we do not insist that formulas must contain taurine. This is an area of active investigation which bears close observation.

GUIDELINES

Human milk

Human milk fed at 185–200 ml per kg will provide an empirically 'safe' (albeit not theoretically optimal) intake of protein during the first weeks of life. There are advantages, particularly for the very LBW baby (< 1500g), if all or part of the milk is fresh and from his own mother. If there is reason to suspect relative protein deficiency (e.g. poor weight gain, very low plasma urea, low plasma prealbumin, nitrogen content of breast milk less than 200 mg/dl), milk may be supplemented with protein or with formula.

Formulas

A formula should not normally contain less than 1.5 g per dl and 2.25 g per 100 kcal when fed at 130 kcal per kg (2.9 g protein per kg.day). If a formula containing 2.25 g per 100 kcal was fed at less than 130 kcal per kg then the protein intake may be too low.

Formulas with a protein:energy ratio as high as 3.1 g per 100 kcal should be used with caution at all times and at present are not recommended when the total energy intake exceeds 130 kcal per kg (4 g of protein per kg per day). Between these figures it is difficult to give more specific guidelines.

The amino acid content of the protein in the formula should not fall below that of breast milk. Lysine availability should be as high as possible and lysine blockage products as low as possible but more precise guidelines cannot be given (see Chapter 17). A specific recommendation about taurine supplementation is not made until there is definite *clinical* evidence of benefit. Similarly, precise guidelines on the whey:casein ratio cannot be given; at present all LBW formulas are whey predominant; this may change in the future but currently there is no compelling evidence to do so.

REFERENCES

1. Ziegler E.E., Biga R.L. & Fomon S.J. (1981). Nutritional requirements of premature infants. In: *Pediatric Nutrition* (Ed. R.M. Suskind) pp. 29–39. Raven Press, New York.
2. Gordon H.H., Levine S.Z. & McNamara H. (1947). Feeding of premature infants: A comparison of human and cow's milk. *Am. J. Dis. Child.* 73, 442–52.
3. Young W.F., Poynet-Wale P., Hymphreys H., Finch E. & Broadbent I. (1950). Protein requirements in infants. 3. The nutrition of premature infants. *Arch. Dis. Child.* 25, 31–51.
4. Omans W.B., Barness L.A., Rose C S. & György P. (1961). Prolonged feeding studies in premature infants. *J. Pediatr.* 59, 951–7.
5. Crosse V.M., Hickmans E.M., Haworth B.E. & Aubrey J. (1954). The value of human milk compared with other feeds for premature infants. *Arch. Dis. Child.* 29, 178.
6. Levin B., Mackay H.M.M., Neil C.A., Oberholzer V.G. & Whitehead T.P. (1959). Weight gains, serum protein levels, and health of breast fed and artificially fed infants. *Spec. Rep. Ser. Med. Res. Coun.* 296, 115. HMSO, London.
7. Davies D.P. (1977) Adequacy of expressed breast milk for early growth of preterm infants. *Arch. Dis. Child.* 52,296.
8. Järvenpää A-L, Räihä N.C.R., Rassin D.K. & Gaull G.E. (1983). Preterm infants fed human milk attain intrauterine weight gain. *Acta Paediatr. Scand.* 72, 239–43.
9. Räihä N.C.R., Heinonen K., Rassin D.K. & Gaull G.E. (1976). Milk protein quality and quantity in low-birth-weight infants: I. Metabolic responses and effects on growth. *Pediatrics* 57, 659–74.
10. Davies D.P. & Evans T.S. (1978). Nutrition and early growth of preterm infants. *Early Hum. Dev.* 2, 383.
11. Scott P.H., Berger H.M. & Wharton B.A. (1985). Growth velocity and plasma amino acids in the newborn. *Pediatr. Res.* 5, 446–50.
12. Senterre J. (1979). Nitrogen balances and protein requirements of the preterm infants. In:

Nutrition and Metabolism of Fetus and Infant (Ed. H.K.A. Visser) pp 195–212. Martinus Nijhoff, The Hague.

13. Berger H.M., Scott P.H., Kenward C., Scott P. & Wharton B.A. (1979). Curd and whey proteins in the nutrition of low birth weight babies. *Arch. Dis. Child.* **54**, 98–104.

14. Atkinson S.A., Bryan M.H. & Anderson G.N. (1981). Human milk feeding in premature infants: protein, fat and carbohydrate balance in the first two weeks of life. *J. Pediatr.* **99**, 617–24.

15. Jackson A.A., Shaw J.C.L., Barber A. & Golden M.H.N. (1981). Nitrogen metabolism in preterm infants fed human donor breast milk: the possible essentiality of glycine. *Pediatr. Res.* **15**, 1454–61.

16. Senterre J. & Rigo J. (1981). Protein requirements of the low birth-weight infants. In: *Physiological and Biochemical Basis for Perinatal Medicine.* (Ed. M. Monset-Covehard and A. Minkowski). S. Karger, Basel.

17. Seashore J.H., Huszar G. & David E.M. (1981). Urinary B-methylhistidine/creatinine ratio as a clinical tool: correlation between B-methylhistidine excretion and metabolic and clinical states in healthy and stressed premature infants. *Metabolism* **70**, 959–69.

18. Shenai J.P., Reynolds J.W. & Babson S.S. (1980). Nutritional balance studies in very low birthweight infants: enhanced nutrient retention rates by an experimental formula. *Pediatrics* **66**, 233–8.

19. Snyderman S.E., Boyer A. Kogut M.D. & Holt L.E. Jr. (1969). The protein requirement of the premature infant. I. The effect of protein intake on the retention of nitrogen. *J. Pediatr.* **74**, 872.

20. Valman H.B., Aikens R., David-Reed Z. & Garrow T.S. (1974). Retention of nitrogen, fat and calories in infants of low birthweight on conventional and high volume feeds. *Brit. Med. J.* **3**, 319.

21. Reichman B., Chessex P., Verellen G., Putet G., Smith J.M., Heim T. & Swyer P.R. (1983). Dietary composition and macronutrient storage in preterm infants. *Pediatrics* **72**, 322–8.

22. Rassin D.K., Gaull G.E., Heinonen K. & Räihä N.C.R. (1977). Milk protein quantity and quality in low-birth-weight infants. II. Effects on selected aliphatic aminoacids in plasma and urine. *Pediatrics* **59**, 407–22.

23. Gaull G.E., Rassin D.K., Räihä N.C.R. & Heinonen K. (1977). Milk protein quantity and quality in low-birth-weight infants. III. Effects on sulfur amino acids in plasma and urine. *J. Pediatr.* **90**, 348–55.

24. Rigo J. & Senterre J. (1977). Is taurine essential for the neonates? *Biol. Neonate* **32**, 73–6.

25. Rassin D.K., Gaull G.E., Räihä N.C.R. & Heinonen K. (1977). Milk protein quantity and quality in low-birth-weight infants. IV. Effects on tyrosine and phenylalanine in plasma and urine. *J. Pediatr.* **90**, 356–60.

26. Rassin D.K., Gaull G.E., Järvenpää A-L. & Räihä N.C.R. (1983). Feeding the low-birthweight infant: II. Effects of taurine and cholesterol supplementation on amino acids and cholesterol. *Pediatrics* **71**, 179–86.

27. Tikanoja J., Simell O., Järvenpää A-L. & Räihä N. (1982). Plasma amino acids in preterm infants after a feed of human milk or formula. *J. Pediatr.* **101**, 248–52.

28. Reichman B.L., Chessex P., Putet G., Verellen G.L.E., Smith J.M., Hein T. & Swyer P.R. (1981). Diet, fat accretion, and growth in premature infants. *N. Engl. J. Med.* **305**, 1495–500.

29. Nicholson J.F. (1970). Rate of protein synthesis in premature infants. *Pediatr. Res.* **4**, 889.

30. Heine W., Plath C., Richter I., Wutzke K. & Töwe J. (1983). ^{14}N-Tracer investigations into the nitrogen metabolism of preterm infants fed mother's milk and a formula diet. *J. Pediatr. Gastroenteral Nutr.* **2**, 606–12.

31. Scott P.H., Berger H.M., Kenward C., Scott P. & Wharton B.A. (1978). Plasma alkaline ribonuclease (EC 3.1.4.22) and nitrogen retention in low birth weight infants. *Br. J. Nutr.* **40**, 459–64.

32. Räihä N.C.R. (1980). Protein in the nutrition of the preterm infant. Biochemical and

nutritional considerations. *Adv. Nutr. Res.* **3**, 173–206.

33. Svenningsen N.W., Lindroth M. & Lindquist B. (1982). Growth in relation to protein intake of low birth weight infants. *Early Hum. Dev.* **6**, 47–58.

34. McIntosh N., Rodeck C.H. & Heath R. (1984). Plasma amino acids of the mid trimester human fetus. *Biol. Neonate* **45**, 218–24.

35. Cockburn F., Giles M., Robins S.P. & Forfar J.O. *J. Obst. Gynaecol. Br. Cwlth* **80**, 10–15.

36. Ginsburg B.E., Lindblad B.S., Lundsjö A., Persson B. & Zetterström R. (1984). Plasma valine and urinary C-peptide in breast fed and artificially fed infants up to 6 months of age. *Acta Paediatr. Scand.* **73**, 213–17.

37. Borch-Johnsen K., Mandrup-Poulsen T., Zachau-Christiansen B., Joner G., Christy M., Kastrup K. & Nerup J. (1984). Relation between breast-feeding and incidence rates of insulin-dependent diabetes mellitus. *Lancet* (November) **10**, 1083–6.

38. Young V.R. (1981). Protein-energy interrelationships in the newborn: a brief consideration of some basic aspects. In: *Textbook of Gastroenterology and Nutrition in Infancy* (Ed. E. Lebenthal). Vol. 1, pp 257–63. Raven Press, New York.

39. Bezkorovairy A. (1977). Human milk and colostrum proteins: a review. *J. Dairy Sci.* **60**, 1023–37.

40. Jenness R. (1979). The composition of human milk. *Sem. Perinatol.* **3**, 225–39.

41. Räihä N.C.R. (1985). Nutritional proteins in milk and the protein requirement of normal infants. *Pediatrics* **75**, 136–42.

42. Hambraeus L. (1977). Proprietary milk versus human breast milk in infant feeding. *Pediatr. Clin. North Am.* **24**, 17–36.

43. Atkinson B.A., Bryan M.J. & Anderson G.H. (1978). Human milk: difference in nitrogen concentration in milk from mothers of term and premature infants. *J. Pediatr.* **93**, 67–9.

44. Gross S.J., David R.J., Bauman L. & Tomarelli R.M. (1980). Nutritional composition of milk produced by mothers delivering preterm. *J. Pediatr.* **96**, 641–4.

45. Butte N.F., Gazra C., Johnson C.A., Smith E.O. & Nichols B.L. (1984). Longitudinal changes in milk composition of mothers delivering preterm and term infants. *Early Hum. Dev.* **9**, 153–62.

46. Hibberd C.M., Brooke O.G., Carter N.D., Hong M. & Harzer G. (1982). Variation in the composition of breast milk during the first 5 weeks of lactation: Implications for the feeding of preterm infants. *Arch. Dis. Child.* **57**, 658–62.

47. Sann L., Bienven J., Bienven F., Lahet C. & Bethenod M. (1981). Comparison of the composition of breast milk from mothers of term and preterm infants. *Acta Paediatr. Scand.* **70**, 115–16.

48. Anderson D., Pittard W., Shulman P., Mitman F., Merkatz R. & Kerr D. (1981). Comparative nutrient composition of human milk. *Pediatr. Res.* **15**, 525.

49. Lucas A., Lucas P.J., Chavin S.I., Lyter R.L.J. & Baum J.D. (1980). A human milk formula. *Early Hum. Dev.* **4/1**, 15–18.

50. Hagelberg S., Lindblad B.S., Lundsjö A., Carlsson B., Fonden R., Fujita H., Lassfolk G. & Lindqvist B. (1982). The protein tolerance of very low weight infants fed human milk protein enriched mother's milk. *Acta Paediatr. Scand.* **71**, 597–601.

51. Hylmö P., Polberger S., Axelsson A., Jakobsson I. & Räihä N. (1984). Preparation of fat and protein from banked human milk: Its use in feeding very-low-birth-weight infants. In: *Human Milk Banking* (eds A.F. Williams & J.D. Baum) pp 55–61. Nestlé Nutrition Workshop. Raven Press, New York.

52. Järvenpää A-L., Räihä N.C.R., Rassin D.K. & Gaull G.E. (1983). Feeding the low-birth-weight infant: I. Taurine and cholesterol supplementation of formula does not affect growth and metabolism. *Pediatrics* **71**, 171–8.

53. Valman H.B., Brown R.J.K., Palmer T., Oberholtzer V.G. & Levin B. (1971). Protein intake and plasma amino acids of infants of low birth weight. *Br. Med. J.* **4**, 789–91.

54. American Academy of Pediatrics Committee on Nutrition (1977). Nutritional needs of

low-birth-weight infants. *Pediatrics* **60**, 519–30.

55. Järvenpää A-L. (1983). Feeding the low-birth-weight infant: IV: Fat absorption as a function of diet and duodenal bile acids. *Pediatrics* **72**, 684–9.

56. Watkins J.B., Järvenpää A-L., Szczepanik Van-Leeuven P., Kein P.D., Rassin D.K., Gaull G.E. & Räihä N.C.R. (1983). Feeding the low-birth-weight infant: V. Effects of human milk, taurine and cholesterol on bile acid kinetics. *Gastroenterology* **85**, 793–800.

57. Järvenpää A-L., Rassin D.K., Kuitunen P., Gaull G.E. & Räihä N.C.R. (1983). Feeding the low-birth-weight infant: III. Diet influences bile acid metabolism. *Pediatrics* **72**, 677–83.

58. Putet G., Senterre J., Rigo J. & Salle B. (1984). Nutrient balance, energy utilization, and composition of weight gain in very-low-birth-weight infants fed pooled human milk or a preterm formula. *J. Pediatr.* **105**, 79–85.

59. Hernell O. (1975). Human milk lipases. III. Physiological implications of bile salt stimulated lipase. *Eur. J. Clin. Invest.* **5**, 267–70.

60. Gross S.J. (1981). Growth and metabolic response of preterm infants fed preterm and mature breast milk. *Pediatr. Res.* **15**, 523.

61. Pearce J.L. & Buchanan L.F. (1979). Breast milk and breast feeding in very low-birth-weight infants. *Arch. Dis. Child.* **54**, 897–9.

62. Rigo J. & Senterre J. (1980). Optimal threonine intake for preterm infants on oral or parenteral nutrition. *J. Parent. Enter. Nutr.* **4**, 15–17.

63. Brueton M.J., Berger H.M., Brown G.A., Ablitt L., Iyngkaran N. & Wharton B.A. (1978). Duodenal bile acid conjugation pattern and dietary sulphur amino acids in the newborn. *Gut* **19**, 95–100.

5
Fat

NUTRITIONAL BACKGROUND

General

Fat provides about half the energy in the diet of the milk fed infant. Adequate energy intakes are unlikely to be achieved if the fat content falls much below 30% of the total energy. Absorbed fat is disposed of in three ways:

1   As an energy source, by the metabolism of free fatty acids or ketone bodies in the tissues.

2   As an energy store, by the deposition of triglyceride in adipose tissue.

3   As essential components of all tissues, but particularly of the central nervous system (1).

Variable amounts of fat are excreted in the faeces, a greater proportion of the intake being lost in preterm than in full term infants (2–8).

Essential Fatty Acids (EFA)

EFA are a group of naturally occurring unsaturated fatty acids of chain length 18, 20 or 22 C atoms and containing 2–6 double bonds in CIS-configuration. The basic EFA are linoleic and ∝-linolenic acids. Others are derived from these, including arachidonic and docosahexaenoic acids. There is evidence that there may be active transport of these across the placenta, since their concentrations in cord blood are higher than in maternal blood (9). However, cord blood concentrations of linoleic acid are always lower than in maternal blood, and are lower in immature than in mature infants (9). The essential nature of these fatty acids is related to their role as components of phospholipids and as precursors of prostaglandins and leukotrienes (10–12).

Other fats and related compounds

Cholesterol
Breast-fed infants tend to have higher concentrations of serum cholesterol than

formula-fed infants. This is discussed in the ESPGAN guidelines on Infant Nutrition. The same is true for preterm infants (13). Plasma cholesterol concentrations are reduced when the intake of polyunsaturated fatty acids is high (14). The significance of these findings in the long term is unknown, but may have relevance to the use of adapted formulas for preterm infants. Formulas containing vegetable oils are rich in phytosterols and three to fivefold increases in plasma phytosterols occur in infants fed such formulas (15). The implication of this in the long term is unknown, but infants on phytosterol-rich diets have phytosterols incorporated into aortic tissue (16).

Carnitine

Carnitine is a quarternary amine (β-hyroxy--trimethylamino butyric acid) which has an important function in the metabolism of lipids in mammalian tissues. Its role is to facilitate the transport of long chain fatty acids across the mitochondrial membrane (17,18). It is synthesized in the body (17) and there is evidence that synthesis may be deficient in preterm infants (19). Plasma and tissue concentrations fall in infants with deficient carnitine intake, for example on total parenteral nutrition (19,20) but the implications of this are uncertain. It has been reported that underweight infants show increased weight gain if fed a carnitine-supplemented diet (21,22). A full term infant with symptoms apparently due to carnitine deficiency has been described (23) but there is no evidence as yet to suggest that preterm infants suffer clinical illness as a result of deficient carnitine intake. Carnitine is present both in breast milk (total carnitine 39–63 μM/1) and in cow's milk based formulas (total carnitine 60–90 μM/1) (24). Plasma concentrations of orally fed infants rise after birth (25).

Choline

Choline is the base of phosphatidyl choline, a phospholipid whose usual fatty acid components are oleic and palmitic acid. It is the precursor of acetycholine and thus quite high concentrations are present in the central nervous system. The brain is probably not capable of synthesizing choline and depends on circulating choline for its supply. About half the circulating choline is of dietary origin (26) and brain choline and ACH concentrations vary with the dietary intake of choline (27). Maternal choline deficiency produces hypertension in the offspring of rats (28). A human deficiency state is not recognized. It is likely that adequate choline is supplied in milk whether it is of human or bovine origin.

In utero accumulation

Few data are available on fetal fat accumulation. Data of Widdowson & Spray (29) and Kelly *et al.* (30) suggest that fat storage is minimal until about 26 weeks gestation (when total body fat amounts to about 1% of body weight) and that by term it accounts for 10–20% of body weight. Assuming that the body of the term neonate weighing 3500 g contains 16% by weight of fat, the total fat accumulation from 26 weeks to term amounts to 550 g (4960 kcal). Most of this fat is probably derived from *de novo* synthesis in fetal tissues (31,32), although free fatty acids and particularly EFA are transported across the placenta (33). There is no good evidence that there is a critical period for the development of the adipocyte or its storage capacity. Adipocytes are small in preterm infants of all gestations, and increase in size and number postnatally (34). Body stores of EFA are lower in preterm than in term infants and both adipose tissue and plasma liquids in the fetus show reduced concentrations of polyunsaturated fatty acids (11,35).

Limitations on the absorption of fat by preterm infants

Fat absorption in infancy is affected by the type of fat ingested, and by the immaturity of the physiological mechanisms concerned with digestion and absorption. Full-term infants absorb fat less efficiently than adults (36), but preterm infants may have severe steatorrhoea when fed unsuitable formulas (2–5,37).

Type of fat ingested

The efficiency of absorption of fat is affected by the chain length and the degree of saturation of its constituent fatty acids (2,3,5,6,38,39), by the configuration of the triglyceride molecule (40,41), and by the presence of lipases in the milk (42,43).

Chain length and degree of saturation of fatty acids
There is general agreement that human infants absorb long chain fatty acids best if they are unsaturated (2,44,45). About 65% of the long chain fatty acids in the breast milk of western women are unsaturated (mainly C18:1 and C18:2) and are almost completely absorbed by the infant. On the other hand bovine milk has a high proportion of C16:0, which is less well absorbed, and saturated long chain fatty acids form two-thirds of its fat content (46). This is likely to be the principal reason for the relatively poor absorption of cow's milk fat by preterm infants. Vegetable oils, which contain a higher proportion of unsaturated fats, are better absorbed (2,3,5).

Configuration of triglyceride molecule
Fatty acids esterified in the 2-position (β) are less readily hydrolysed by

pancreatic lipase than those in 1- and 3- ($\propto$) positions. This affects the absorption of fat because the monoglyceride of certain fatty acids, e.g. palmitic acid, is more readily absorbed than the free fatty acid (40,41). In human milk about 98% of the lipid is triacyglycerol in which most of the 2-position ester is palmitic acid. Thus the digestion products in the gut contain a high proportion of palmitate monoglyceride which is well absorbed. In bovine milk only about 30% of the palmitate is esterified in the 2-position and it is thus less well absorbed (40,41). This accounts for the high proportion of palmitic acid in the stools of infants fed formulas containing cow's milk fat (48). There is some evidence (49) that palmitate 2-monoglyceride may be less well absorbed than the monopalmitate when bile salt concentrations are low, so the interpretation of results obtained in full term infants may not necessarily apply to the preterm.

Milk lipases
Human milk contains bile-salt stimulated lipase (42,43). There is substantial evidence that this is of major significance in fat digestion. Williamson *et al.* (37) found that absorption was reduced by about 40% when the milk was pasteurized or boiled. Atkinson *et al.* (50) found better fat absorption from raw preterm mother's milk than from pasteurized banked breast milk. Soderhjelm (51), however, found that pasteurization had no effect on fat absorption in preterm infants.

Immaturity of physiological mechanisms

Whatever type of fat is given, some preterm infants show significant fat malabsorption compared with term infants and older children. There are therefore physiological limitations to digestion and absorption which are related to immaturity. Deficiences have been identified in two main areas: (a) pancreatic lipase secretion, and (b) bile salt secretion. There has been recent interest in lingual lipase which, if deficient, may also be a limiting factor in fat absorption. There is no evidence that the mucosol phase of fat absorption is unsatisfactory in preterm infants.

Pancreatic lipase secretion
Preterm infants have reduced pancreatic response to secretin and pancreozymin-cholecystokinin (52), low lipase activity in duodenal juice (53,54) and increased concentrations of duodenal triglycerides (53), compared with more mature infants.

Bile salt secretion
Duodenal bile acid concentrations are often well below critical micellar

concentrations in preterm infants (56,57). Watkins *et al.* (58) have shown that this is due to a reduction in bile acid pool size and synthesis rate, which are reduced to 30–50% of the values found at term. Järvenpää *et al.* (59) found that duodenal concentrations on conjugated bile acids and bile acid pool size were greater in preterm infants fed human milk than in those fed cow's milk formulas, but there was no significant increase in the concentrations with time on any type of feeding during the first 5 weeks of life. Infants fed breast milk have mainly taurine conjugated bile acids in contrast to formula-fed infants who have mainly glycine conjugation (60), cow's milk being a poor source of taurine. However, the supplementation of formulas with taurine does not improve fat absorption in the preterm infants (61).

Lingual lipase

Saliva contains a powerful lipase secreted by the lingual serous glands. Its role in fat digestion is uncertain but some preterm infants are deficient in it (62). It is stimulated by sucking (63), so the tube-fed infant may be at a disadvantage. More work is necessary.

The problems caused by the immaturity of the physiological mechanisms of fat absorption are likely to be aggravated by naso-jejunal feeding.

Interrelationships between fat absorption and the absorption of other nutrients

There are a number of theoretical ways in which fat malabsorption may be associated with the detrimental malabsorption of other nutrients.

Vitamin absorption

Fat malabsorption is associated with malabsorption of vitamin E in preterm infants (64), but Morales *et al.* (65) found that varying the fat intake had no effect on vitamin A absorption and vitamin D given in a dose of 100 iu/day to healthy preterm infants is probably well absorbed (66).

Mineral absorption

Katz & Hamilton (55) found that calcium supplements depressed fat absorption by preterm infants, but this effect was not shown in Barltroop's studies (4). A number of studies have demonstrated that calcium malabsorption by preterm infants seems to be independent of fat malabsorption (4,37,41,67). However calcium soaps are sometimes formed in the gut causing fat bolus obstruction (68).

Protein retention

Nitrogen appears to improve with improved fat absorption (6,37). This is likely to be a general effect of the improved energy balance which allows better growth.

AVAILABLE FOODS

Manipulations of the fat composition of infant formulas are among the most common sources of variation between formulas. Thus many different forms of dietary fat have been made available for infants, and these have often been insufficiently evaluated. However, formulas are available which contain butter fat alone, blends of butter fat, with various vegetable oils, vegetable oils alone, and blends of vegetable oils and medium chain triglycerides (See Table 1.1).

REQUIREMENTS, ADVISABLE INTAKES

The principal difficulty about making recommendations on the feeding of fat to preterm infants is the lack of data. In eleven studies of fat absorption in such infants in which gestational age is documented and methodology and statistical analyses are well described (4–6,37,50,55,57,67,69–71) the total number of infants studied amounts to 180.

These studies were performed using EBM and 14 formulas of varying composition, giving an average of 12 infants per type of feed. Taking account of varying gestation and postnatal age, the data are very scanty indeed and there is little reliable information about growth in relation to fat retention.

Qualitative and quantitative requirements

Qualitative

Essential fatty acids
   (a) *Lower limit.* Preterm infants may be more vulnerable than full term infants to EFA deficiency because:
1   They suffer fat malabsorption.
2   They may be growing rapidly.
3   They have little adipose tissue and therefore may have only small reserves of EFA.
Various authors (72–75) have studied EFA requirements in infants and showed that clinical and histological evidence of EFA deficiency may occur when linoleic acid forms less than 1% of total dietary energy (~100 mg per 100 kcal). When there is a marginal EFA content in the diet, a low caloric intake

and slow growth are less likely to be associated with clinical deficiency than a high caloric intake and rapid growth (11). Recommendations for minimum intake of EFA in full term infants have thus generally allowed a safety margin. For example, ESPGAN, Codex Alimentarius and French legislation adopted 300 mg per 100 kcal. We feel that preterm infants should be allowed an even greater safety margin and recommend a minimum intake of 500 mg per 100 kcal (~4.5% of total calories). It is possible that deficiency of linolenic acid or inhibition of its formation may sometimes occur (76), so we recommend that not less than 55 mg per 100 kcal (~0.5% of total calories), be provided in this form.

(b) *Upper limit*. Linoleic acid in breast milk may, in extreme cases, vary from 1–22% of total fat (0.6–1.3 g per 100 kcal) depending on the mother's diet (77). The European range is about 7–12% of total fat (0.4–0.7 g per 100 kcal). It is therefore not sensible to make tight recommendations. However, very high intakes (>20% or 1.2 g/100 kcal) should probably be avoided because of the possibility of impaired immune responses (78).

Cholesterol, carnitine, choline
There are no recommendations on the desirable level of intake of these nutrients.

Fatty acids composition and absorption
Longer chain unsaturated fatty acids (C12 and above) are better absorbed than saturated fatty acids of the same chain length, and thus there should be a predominance of unsaturated fatty acids in a formula for preterm infants. Vegetable fat is not necessarily superior to fats of animal origin but is acceptable. There is no basis for any recommendations to limit the amount of C12 in formulas since it is atherogenic in rats (79), but we do not feel that there is enough evidence to give rise to concern in human infant feeding. The use of medium chain triglycerides is discussed below.

Quantitative

Minimum total fat intake is determined by the tolerated intake of protein and CHO at a given energy level. Hence at an energy intake of 130 kcal/kg per day and allowing a maximum protein energy of 12% (3 g/100 kcal) and maximum CHO energy of 56% (14 g/100 kcal), fat will provide 32% of the dietary energy (4.7 g/kg, 3.6 g/100 kcal). Provision of less fat will result in energy intake below recommended level, or protein/CHO intake above recommended level. If these figures are applied to the minimum recommended energy concentration of 65 kcal/100 ml feed, the minimum fat concentration is 2.3 g/100 ml. This is unusually low and we consider it would be rarely used but would be acceptable if the minimum EFA recommendation was met.

Maximum total fat intake is determined by fat digestibility and the need to avoid gross steatorrhoea, and also possibly by limitations of metabolic utilization. Thus Brooke (80) found that although net energy retention was higher on a fat intake of 10.2 g/kg per day than on 6.2 g/kg per day there was no significant difference in weight gain, probably due to a higher rate of postprandial metabolism. Fat intakes of up to 11 g/kg per day appear to be tolerated by most preterm infants without adverse symptoms (81). There are insufficient data to make recommendations for maximum fat intakes in infants <1000 g but it should not be necessary to exceed 9 g/kg. Fat intakes at minimum and maximum energy intakes and minimum and maximum fat content of feed, are given in Table 5.1.

Table 5.1 Fat recommendations.
Daily fat intake at different energy intakes and fat content of feeds.

Fat content of feed	Minimum 3.6 g/100 kcal	Average 5.3 g/100 kcal	Maximum 7.0 g/100 kcal
Energy intake:			
Minimum (110 kcal/kg per day)	4.0 g/kg	5.8 g/kg	7.7 g/kg
Average (130 kcal/kg per day)	4.7 g/kg	6.9 g/kg	9.1 g/kg
Maximum (165 kcal/kg per day)	5.9 g/kg	8.7 g/kg	11.6 g/kg*

*11.6 g not allowed by our recommendations

Comments on breast milk fat

In almost all studies, fat absorption from EBM has been good in preterm infants, but less good than in term infants. The mean coefficient of fat absorption in 56 infants in various studies is 75% but ranges from 45% to 90%. In only one study (50) has fat absorption from human milk been investigated in very low birth weight (VLBW) infants, within the first 10 days of life, a critical period for energy balance.

Williamson *et al.* (37) found poor fat absorption in seven VLBW infants who were given pasteurized EBM and very poor when they were given boiled EBM. Atkinson *et al.* (50) also found that fat absorption from pooled pasteurized breast milk was worse than from fresh preterm mother's milk. Therefore it is reasonable to assume that the destruction of milk lipase by heat treatment is likely to decrease fat absorption in some infants.

Accepting the adequacy of fat absorption from raw human milk under most circumstances there are two further potential problems relating to its use in preterm infants: (a) the variability of fat content of human milk and (b) the tendency for human milk fat to adhere to receptacles and feeding tubes.

Variations of fat content
The variability of milk fat is enormous. Carroll *et al.* (82) found fat concentrations varying between 5.8 and 67 g/l while Hibbard *et al.* (83) found energy values in the milks of preterm mothers ranging between 45 and 105 kcal/100 ml, a difference largely determined by variations in the fat content. Reasons for variability are largely due to methods of collection. For example, foremilk has a lower fat content than hindmilk, and reflex drip milk, which is used in some nurseries, has a very low fat content (84). Preterm mother's milk collected under standardized conditions shows greater variability than full term milk (83). Thus some way of monitoring fat intake is essential in babies fed EBM if an accurate knowledge of energy intake is required.

Adherence of milk fat to containers
It should be remembered that significant losses of human milk fat may occur during feeding on account of its tendency to adhere to the walls of tubing and containers, particularly glass ones (85).

Comments on formulas

There is general agreement in the literature that formulas containing cow's milk as the sole or principal form of fat are less well digested by the preterm infant than those containing vegetable oils or medium chain triglycerides (2,3,5,6,51,63,86). In various studies the mean coefficient of fat absorption from cow's milk fat formulas was 53%, compared with 72% from formulas containing vegetable oils. There is therefore no justification for the use of cow's milk fat as the sole fat in formulas fed to preterm infants. It is less easy to determine from the literature what the 'ideal' fat composition of such formulas should be. Many different vegetable oils have been used in attempts to reproduce the fatty acid composition of human milk and from the point of view of efficiency of absorption, there seems little to choose between them. However, formulas containing high concentrations of C16:0 in the α-positions are significantly less well absorbed than those with low concentrations (41,70). All new formulas should be tested for fat absorption.

Four studies have shown better net fat absorption from formulas containing MCT (C8,10) (6,47,87,88). These studies showed an improvement in fat absorption of about 20% but with only small differences in weight gain. A formula containing 80% of fat as MCT gave little advantage over one containing 40% (47). Brooke (80), using MCT supplements to a vegetable oil formula, found only marginally better energy balance and no significant differences in weight gain. There is no evidence that MCT are harmful but little is known about their long term effects on growth or metabolism and it is possible that they are incorporated into myelin. It is therefore prudent to be cautious and formulas containing more than 40% of fat as MCT are not recommended.

SUMMARY OF RECOMMENDATIONS

Breast milk fat

1   Fat is well absorbed from raw human milk by preterm infants but not necessarily better than from a well-designed formula. When human milk fat is heated, there is some loss of lipolytic activity but there are insufficient data to make recommendations about the optimal processing. To ensure the best fat absorption, human milk should be given raw.
2   Human milk fat content is extremely variable and thus should be monitored if there is inadequate weight gain. Reflex drip milk is particularly low in fat.
3   Human milk tends to separate and adhere to containers. This results in a reduction of the energy density of the milk, especially when it is administered by continuous infusion. This can be minimized by agitating the container or arranging for infusion syringes to discharge in an upward direction, so that any separated fat is given first.

Formulas

Qualitative

Fatty acid composition. It is difficult to make definitive recommendations about the fat composition of formulas for preterm infants. A number of blends of vegetable and animal fats have been used successfully. In general, longer chain unsaturated fatty acids (C12 and above) are better absorbed than saturated fatty acids of the same chain length and thus there should be a predominance of unsaturated fatty acids in a formula for preterm infants. Vegetable fat is not necessarily superior to fats of animal origin but is acceptable. We do not feel it necessary to stipulate a minimum content of animal fats. Formulas containing more than 40% of fat as MCT are not recommended.

Essential fatty acids. Linoleic acid should account for at least 4.5% of total calories (0.5 g per 100 kcal). We are aware that some formulas contain an EFA content greater than 20% of total fat. This is higher than is found in breast milk and we feel there should be no need for such a high proportion. We suggest an upper limit of 20% of total fatty acid (1.2 g/100 kcal). Linolenic acid should account for at least 0.5% of total calories (55 mg per 100 kcal).

Carnitine, cholesterol and choline. We are unable to make recommendations about the desirable intake of these nutrients in preterm infants.

Quantitative

The minimum intake of fat is determined by the need to provide adequate dietary energy and to limit the maximum intake of CHO and protein.

At the average recommended energy intake of 130 kcal/kg per day and allowing the maxium recommended intakes of CHO and protein, fat intake will be 4.7 g/kg (3.6 g/100 kcal).

At the minimum recorded energy intake of 110 kcal/kg per day and again allowing the maxium recommended intakes of CHO and protein, fat intake will be 4.0 g/kg. This fat intake is unnecessarily low but would be acceptable provided that the requirements for EFA were met.

The maximum intake of fat relates to the capacity for absorption. Although fat intakes of up to 11 g/kg daily have been shown to be tolerated by some small preterm infants, we consider it unnecessary to give fat intakes in excess of 9 g/kg or to exceed a fat density of 7.0 g/100 kcal in a formula.

REFERENCES

1. Crawford M.A. (1976). Lipids and the development of the human brain. *Biochem. Soc. Trans.* **4**, 231.
2. Tidwell H.C., Holt L.E., Farrow H.L. & Neal S. (1935). Studies in fat metabolism. *J. Pediatr.* **6**, 481.
3. Davidson M. & Bauer C.H. (1960). Patterns of fat excretion in premature infants fed various preparations of milk. *Pediatrics* **25**, 375.
4. Barltrop D. & Oppé T.E. (1973). Calcium and fat absorption by low birthweight infants from a calcium-supplemented milk formula. *Arch Dis. Child.* **48**, 580.
5. Barltrop D. & Oppé T.E. (1973). Absorption of fat and calcium by low birthweight infants from milks containing butterfat and olive oil. *Arch. Dis. Child.* **48**, 496.
6. Roy C.C., Ste-Marie M., Chartrand R.T., Weber A., Bard H. & Doray B. (1975). Correction of the malabsorption of the preterm infant with a medium-chain triglyceride formula. *J. Pediatr.* **86**, 446.
7. Welsch H., Heinz F., Legally G. & Stuhlfauth K. (1965). Fettresorption aus Frauenmilch bei Neugeborenen. *Kiln. Wochenschr.* **43**, 902.

8. Widdowson E.M. (1965). Absorption and excretion of fat, nitrogen and minerals from 'filled' milks by babies one week old. *Lancet* **ii**, 1099.
9. Friedman Z., Danon A., Lamberth E.L. *et al.* (1978). Cord blood fatty acid composition in infants and in their mothers during the third trimester. *J. Pediatr.* **92**, 461.
10. Crawford M.A., Sinclair A.J., Msuya P.M. & Munhambo A. (1973). Structural lipids and their polyenoic constituents in breast milk. In: *Dietary Lipids and Postnatal Development* (ed. C. Galli, G. Jacini & A. Recile) Raven Press, New York.
11. Friedman Z. (1979). Polyunsaturated fatty acids in the low-birth-weight infant. *Sem. Perinatol.* **3**, 341.
12. Rankin J.A., Hitchcock M., Merrill W., Bach M.K., Brashler J.R. & Askenase P.W. (1982). IgE dependent release of leukotriene C4 from alveolar macrophages. *Nature* **297**, 329.
13. Rassin D.K., Gaull G.E., Järvenpää A-L & Räihä N.C.R. (1983). Feeding the low-birth-weight infant: II. Effects of taurine and cholesterol supplementation on aminoacids and cholesterol. *Pediatrics* **71**, 179.
14. Van Biervliet J.P., Vinaimont N., Caster H. *et al.* (1981). Plasma apoprotein and lipid patterns in newborns. *Acta Paediat. Scand.* **70**, 851.
15. Mellies M., Glueck C.J., Sweeney C., Fallat R.W., Tsang R.C. & Ishikawa T.T. (1976). Plasma and dietary phytosterols in children. *Pediatrics* **88**, 914.
16. Mellies M., Ishikawa T.T., Glueck C.J., Bove K. & Morrison J. (1976). Phytosterols in aortic tissue in adults and infants. *J. Lab. Clin. Med.* **88**, 914.
17. Mitchell M.E. (1978). Carnitine metabolism in human subjects. 1. Normal metabolism. *Am. J. Clin. Nutr.* **31**, 293.
18. Bressler R. & Katz R.I. (1965). The role of carnitine in acetoacetate production and fatty acid synthesis. In: *Recent Research in Carnitine* (ed. G. Wolf) M I T Press, Cambridge.
19. Penn D., Schmidt-Sommerfeld E. & Pascu F. (1981). Decreased tissue carnitine concentrations in newborn infants receiving total parenteral nutrition. *J. Pediatr.* **98**, 976.
20. Schiff D., Chan G., Seccomb D. & Hahn P. (1979). Plasma carnitine levels during intravenous feeding of the neonate. *J. Pediatr.* **95**, 1043.
21. Alexander F., Peeters H. & Vuylsteke P. (1958). Activite clinique et metabolique de lar carnitine chez l'enfant. In: *Proteides of the Biological Fluids.* pp 306–10. Proceedings of the 6th Colloquim, Bruges. Elsevier, Amsterdam.
22. Borniche P. & Canlorbe P. (1960). Action clinique et humorale de la carnitine dan les syndromes de denutrition post-infectieux de l'enfance. *Clin. Chim. Acta* **5**, 171.
23. Slonim A.E., Borum P.R., Tanaka K. *et al.* (1981). Dietary dependent carnitine deficiency as a cause of non-ketotic hypoglycemia in an infant. *J. Pediatr.* **99**, 551.
24. Novak M., Wieser P.B., Buch M. & Hahn P. (1979). Acetylcarnitine and free carnitine in body fluids before and after birth. *Pediatr. Res.* **13**, 10.
25. Novak M., Monkus E.F., Chung D. & Buch M. (1981). Carnitine in the perinatal metabolism of lipids. *Pediatrics* **67**, 95.
26. Hanin I. & Schuberth J. (1974). Labelling of acetylcholine in the brain of mice fed on a diet containing deuterium labelled choline. *J. Neurochem.* **23**, 819.
27. Nagler A.L., Dettbarn W.D., Seifter E. & Levenson S.M. (1968). Tissue levels of acetylcholine and acetylcholinesterase in weanling rats subjected to acute choline deficiency. *J. Nutr.* **94**, 13.
28. Hurley L.S. (1980). *Developmental Nutrition*, p. 164. Prentice Hall, New York.
29. Widdowson E.M. & Spray C.M. (1951). Chemical development *in utero*. *Arch Dis. Child.* **26**, 205.
30. Kelly H.J., Sloan R.E. Hoffman W. & Saunders C. (1951). Accumulation of nitrogen and six minerals in the human fetus during gestation. *Human Biol.* **23**, 61.
31. Hursch J., Farguhar J., Ahrens E.H., Peterson M.L. & Stoffel W. (1960). Studies of adipose

tissues in man; a microtechnique for sampling and analysis. *Am J. Clin Nutr.* **8**, 499.

32. Dancis J., Jansen V., Kayden H.J., Schneider H. & Levitz M. (1973). Transfer across perfused human placenta II: Free fatty acids. *Pediatr. Res.* **7**, 192.
33. Whaley W.H., Zuspan F.P. & Nelson G.H. (1968). Correlation between maternal and fetal plasma levels of glucose and free fatty acids. *Am. J. Obstet. Gynecol.* **105**, 670.
34. Bonnet F.P. (ed) (1981). *Adipose Tissue in Childhood.* C R C Press, Florida.
35. Fosbrooke A.S. & Wharton B.A. (1973). Plasma lipids in umbilical cord blood from infants of normal and low birth weight. *Biol. Neonate* **23**, 330.
36. Grand R.J., Sutphen J.L. & Montgomery R.K. (1979). The immature intestine: implications for nutrition of the neonate. In: *Development of Mammalian Absorptive Processes.* Ciba Foundation Symposium No. 70. Excerpta Medica, Amsterdam.
37. Williamson S., Finucane E., Ellis H. & Gamsu H.R. (1978). Effect of heat treatment of human milk on absorption of nitrogen, fat, sodium, calcium and phosphorus by preterm infants. *Arch Dis. Child.* **53**, 555.
38. Williams M.L., Rose C.S., Morrow G., Sloan S.E. & Barness L.A. (1970). Calcium and fat absorption in the neonatal period. *Am. J. Clin. Nutr.* **23**, 1322.
39. Fomon S.J., Ziegler E.E., Thomas L.N., Jensen R.L. & Filer L.J. (1970). Excretion of fat by normal full-term infants fed various milks and formulas *Am. J. Clin. Nutr.* **23**, 1299.
40. Tomarelli R.M., Meyer B.J., Weaber J.R. & Bernhardt F.W. (1968). Effect of positional distribution on the absorption of fatty acids of human milk and infant formulas. *J. Nutr.* **95**, 583.
41. Filer R.J., Mattson F.H. & Fomon S.J. (1969). Triglyceride configuration and fat absorption by the human infant. *J. Nutr.* **99**, 293.
42. Frendenberg E. (1953). *Die Frauenmilch-Lipase.* Karger, Basel.
43. Fredikzon B., Hernell O., Blackberg L. & Olivecrona T. (1978). Bile-stimulated lipase in human milk. *Pediatr. Res.* **12**, 1048.
44. Holt L.E., Tidwell H.C., Kirk C.M., Cross D.M. & Neale S. (1935). Fat absorption in normal infants. *J. Pediatr.* **6**, 427.
45. Widdowson E.M. (1974). Nutrition. In: *Scientific Foundations of Paediatrics* (eds J. Davis & J. Dobbing). Heinemann, London.
46. Jensen R.G., Hagerty M.M. & McMahon K.E. (1978). Lipids of human milk and infant formulas: a review. *Am. J. Clin. Nutr.* **31**, 990.
47. Tantibhedhyangkul P. & Hashim S. (1971). Clinical and physiological aspects of medium-chain triglycerides. *Bull. N.Y. Acad. Med.* **47**, 17.
48. Hanna F.M., Navarrete D.A. & Hsu F.A. (1970). Calcium-fatty acid absorption in term infants fed human milk and prepared formulas stimulating human milk. *Pediatrics* **45**, 216.
49. Hofman A.F. (1963). The behaviour and solubility of monoglycerides in dilute, miceller bile-salt solution. *Biochem. Biophys. Acta* **70**, 306.
50. Atkinson S.A., Bryan M.H. & Anderson G.H. (1981). Human milk feeding in premature infants: protein, fat and carbohydrate balances in the first two weeks of life. *J. Pediatr.* **99**, 617.
51. Soderhjelm L. (1952). Influence of heat treatment on milk on fat retention by premature infants. *Acta Paediatr. Scand.* **41**, 207.
52. Zoppi G., Andreotti G., Pajo-Ferrara F., Njai D.M. & Gaburro D. (1972). Exocrine pancreatic function in premature and full-term neonates. *Pediatr. Res.* **6**, 880.
53. Geschwind Von R. (1950). Das Verhalten de Pancreasenzyme bei Fruhgebornen. *Ann. Pediatr.* **157**, 176.
54. Lebenthal E. & Lee P.C. (1980). Development of functional response in human exocrine pancreas. *Pediatrics* **66**, 556.
55. Katz L. & Hamilton J.R. (1974). Fat absorption in infants of birthweight less than 1300 g. *J. Pediatr.* **85**, 608.

56. Norman A., Strandvik B. & Ojamae O. (1972). Bile acids and pancreatic enzymes during absorption in the newborn. *Acta Paediatr. Scand.* **61**, 571.
57. Signer E., Murphy G.M., Edkins S. & Anderson C.M. (1974). Role of bile salts in fat malabsorption of premature infants. *Arch Dis. Child.* **49**, 174.
58. Watkins J.B., Szczepanik P., Gould J.B., Klein P. & Lester R. (1975). Bile salt metabolism in the human premature infant. *Gastroenterology* **69**, 706.
59. Järvenpää A-L., Rassin D.K., Kuitunen P., Gaull G.E. & Räihä N.C.R. (1983). Feeding the low-birth-weight infant: III. Diet influences bile acid metabolism. *Pediatrics* **72**, 677
60. Brueton M.J., Berger H.M., Brown G.A., Ablitt- L., Iyngkaran M. & Wharton B.A. (1978). Duodenal bile acid conjugation patterns and dietary sulphur amino acids in the newborn. *Gut* **19**, 35.
61. Watkins J.B., Järvenpää A-L., Szczepanik Van-Leeuwen P., Klein P.D., Räihä N., Rassin D.K. & Gaull G. (1983). Feeding the low birth weight infant: Effects of taurine, cholesterol and human milk on bile acid kinetics. *Gastroenterology* **85**, 793.
62. Hamosh M., Sivasubramanian K.N., Salzman-Mann C. & Hamosh P. (1978). Fat digestion in the stomach of premature infants. *J. Pediatr.* **93**, 674.
63. Hamosh M. (1979). The role of lingual lipase in neonatal fat digestion. In: *Development of Mammalian Absorptive Processes*. Ciba Foundation Symposium No. 70. Excerpta Medica, Amsterdam.
64. Melhorn D.K. & Gross S. (1971). Vitamin E dependent anaemia in the premature infant. *J. Pediatr.* **79**, 581.
65. Morales S., Chung A.W., Lewis J.M., Messian A. & Holt L.E. (1950). Absorption of fat and vitamin A in premature infants. *Pediatrics* **6**, 86.
66. Senterre J. & Salle B. (1982). Calcium and phosphorus economy of the preterm infant and its interaction with vitamin D and its metabolites. *Acta Paediatr. Sand.* (Suppl.) **296**, 85.
67. Shaw J.C. (1976). Evidence for defective skeletal mineralization in low-birth-weight infants: the absorption of calcium and fat. *Pediatrics* **57**, 16.
68. Lewis C.T., Dickson J.A.C. & Swain W.A.J. (1977). Milk bolus obstruction in the neonate. *Arch. Dis. Child.* **52**, 68.
69. Valman H.B., Aitkens R., David-Reed Z. & Garrow J.S. Retention of nitrogen, fat and calories in infants of low birthweight on conventional and high-volume feeds. *Br. Med. J.* **2**, 319.
70. Milner R.D.G., Deodhar Y. Chard C.R. & Grout R.M. (1975). Fat absorption by small babies fed two filled milk formulae. *Arch. Dis. Child.* **50**, 654.
71. Shenai J.P., Jhaveri B.M., Reynolds J.W., Huston R.K. & Babson S.G. (1981). Nutritional balance studies in very low-birthweight infants: role of soy formula. *Pediatrics* **67**, 631.
72. Hansen A.E., Wiese H.F., Boelsche A.N. *et al.* (1963). Role of linoleic acid in infant nutrition: clinical and chemical study of 428 infants fed on milk mixtures varying in kind and amount of fat. *Pediatrics* **31**, 171.
73. Combes M., Pratt E.L. & Wiese H.F. (1962). Essential fatty acids in premature infant feeding. *Pediatrics* **30**, 136.
74. Panos T.C., Stinnett B., Cross E. *et al.* (1961). Metabolic effects of low fat feeding in premature infants. *Fed. Proc.* **20**, 366.
75. Friedman Z., Danon A., Stohlman M. & Oates J. (1976). Rapid onset of essential fatty acid deficiency in the newborn. *Pediatrics* **58**, 640.
76. Holman R.T., Johnson S.B. & Hatch T.F. (1982). A case of human linolenic acid deficiency involving neurological abnormalities. *Am. J. Clin. Nutr.* **35**, 617.
77. Read W.W.C., Lutz P.G. & Tashian A. (1965). Human milk lipids 11. Influence of dietary carbohydrates and fat on the fatty acids of mature milk. A study in four ethnic groups. *Am. J. Clin. Nutr.* **17**, 180.
78. Beisel W.R. (1982) Single nutrients and immunity. *Am. J. Clin. Nutr.* **35**, (Suppl. 2), 417.

79. Wissler R.W. & Vesselinovitch D. (1969). Recent advances in the understanding of the pathogeneses and the revisal of atherosclerosis. *Pathol. Ann.* **4**, 313.

80. Brooke O.G. (1980). Energy balance and metabolic rate in preterm infants fed with standard and high-energy formulas. *Br. J. Nutr.* **44**, 13.

81. Hanmer O.J., Houlsby W.T., Thorn H. *et al.* (1982). Fat as an energy supplement for preterm infants. *Arch. Dis. Child.* **57**, 503.

82. Caroll L., Conlan D. & Davies D.P. (1980). Fat content of banked human milk. *Arch. Dis. Child.* **55**, 969.

83. Hibberd C., Brooke O.G., Carter N.D. & Wood C. (1981). A comparison of protein concentrations and energy in breast milk from preterm and term mothers. *J. Hum. Nutr.* **35**, 189.

84. Lucas A. (1982). Human milk banks. *Lancet* **1**, 103.

85. Brooke O.G. & Barley J. (1978). Loss of energy during continuous infusion of breast milk. *Arch. Dis. Child.* **53**, 344.

86. Zoula J., Melichar V., Novak M., Hann P. & Koldovsky O. (1966). Nitrogen and fat retention in premature infants fed breast milk, 'humanized' cow's milk or half-skimmed milk. *Acta Paediatr. Scand.* **55**, 26.

87. Yamashita F., Shibuya S. & Funatsu I. (1969) Absorption of medium chain triglycerides in low-birth-weight infants. *Kurume Med. J.* **16**, 191.

88. Huston R.K., Reynolds J.W., Jensen C. & Buist N.R.M. (1983). Nutrient and mineral retention and vitamin D absorption in low-birth-weight infants: effect of medium-chain triglycerides. *Pediatrics* **72**, 44.

6
Carbohydrate

NUTRITIONAL BACKGROUND

While carbohydrate is an essential nutrient, lactose itself is not since any galactose which is required for formation of cerebrosides and mucopolysaccharides can be made in the liver from glucose, and children receiving lactose/galactose free diets for many years for the treatment of galactosaemia show normal physical and mental development (1). However, the use of lactose in infant feeding has obvious teleological support and in addition lactose may have certain physiological functions, e.g. enhanced absorption of calcium, magnesium and strontium (2–7) and promotion of the growth of lactobacilli in the intestine (8).

The amount of carbohydrate given to a low birth weight (LBW) baby is closely related to four matters: (a) the prevention of hypoglycaemia; (b) total energy intake required for maintenance and growth; (c) renal solute load of a feed per unit energy and per unit volume of water; (d) intestinal 'tolerance' of the carbohydrate.

Twenty years ago the volumes of milk or formula fed to small babies were increased considerably, so that today hypoglycaemia is less common even in light-for-gestational age babies fed conventional volumes of breast milk or standard formula (e.g. 60 ml/kg per day on the first day increasing to 150 ml/kg per day by day 4, lactose 7.4 g, energy 67 kcal per dl (9,10). LBW babies may require a higher energy intake than normal ones to mimic intrauterine growth or to achieve catch up growth. A simple way of achieving this is to increase the volume of breast milk or a 'standard' formula given to the infant; indeed many paediatricians routinely offer LBW babies 200 ml per kg per day and some much more. However, this approach may be limited mechanically, e.g. due to aspiration or development of a patent ductus arteriosus. Another approach is to increase the strength of the feed offered so that the total energy (and total solids) per unit volume are higher than given to normal babies; increases up to 1.33 times 'normal' strength (i.e. 90 kcal per dl) may be tolerated. This approach is eventually limited by the increase in total solids, perhaps leading to a milk plug, by the increase in the renal solute lead per unit volume, so exceeding the renal concentrating ability, and by increase in the lactose concentration resulting in malabsorption, diarrhoea and acidosis. Caution is therefore necessary. Alternatively, a LBW formula may be used in which, compared to a normal formula, the energy content is increased without increasing lactose concentration, either by adding another well absorbed carbohydrate or by increasing the concentration of fat, or both. These manoeuvres also ensure that renal solute load per unit energy does not rise excessively.

Clearly any other carbohydrate used must be well absorbed. Assessment of carbohydrate absorption is not straightforward, however. The classical balance technique is not appropriate because of the bacterial degradation of carbohydrate in the large intestine, and the other techniques used, e.g. changes in plasma glucose following ingestion, studies of intestinal enzyme activity, measurement of stool carbohydrate and its products, e.g. lactic acid, may give a varying assessment of 'efficiency' of absorption. The enzymes necessary for digestion of maltose and sucrose are well developed in the viable preterm baby [11]. Pancreatic $\propto$-amylase activity is low in young infants [12] so that the use of starch at this age may result in malabsorption, diarrhoea [13] and reduced weight gain in relation to energy intake [7]. Small amounts of pregelatinized starch may be tolerated and apparently absorbed [13,14]. The rise in blood glucose following ingestion of starch is lower but persists far longer [15,16]. Digestion of starch and starch hydrolysates may be explained by the activity of the salivary amylase and the intestinal glucoamylase. This latter enzyme has been shown to be fully developed in the brush border of the intestinal mucosa in neonates. It hydrolyses glucose polymers by the stepwise removal of D-glucose from the non-reducing end of the molecule. It has the greatest affinity for oligosaccharides with 5–9 glucose units [17,18]. Hydrolysates of starch resulting in a mixture of glucose, maltose and glucose polymers are frequently used in infant nutrition, e.g. maltodextrin, corn syrup solids, 'Polycose', 'Caloreen', 'liquid glucose BPC'. They are best defined by their dextrose-equivalent number. A high number indicates more short oligosaccharides and free glucose which may benefit absorption, but also it infers a higher osmolality, which may lead to intestinal intolerance. The rise in blood glucose following the ingestion of corn starch hydrolysate was similar to that following maltose [16] or lactose [19]. However, the insulin response to corn starch hydrolysate was lower than to lactose [19].

AVAILABLE FOODS

Almost all of the carbohydrate in both mature human milk (mean 7.4 g per dl; 11.1 g per 100 kcal) and cow's milk (mean 4.8 g per dl; 7.2 g per 100 kcal) is lactose. The breast milk of mothers delivering preterm babies contains 0.2–0.5

g per dl less. Human milk contains some short chain oligosaccharides, the significance of which is unclear. Most formulas for normal babies contain lactose as the only carbohydrate, but a few also contain other carbohydrate, commonly a glucose polymer such as maltodextrin, occasionally sucrose or starch (total carbohydrate up to 13.0 g per 100 kcal). Formulas specifically designed for LBW babies may contain lactose only (2.3–8.7 g per dl; 2.9–11.6 g per 100 kcal) but most contain lactose together with glucose and/or a glucose polymer (total carbohydrate 6.3–9.7 g per dl; 7.5–12.6 g per 100 kcal see Table 1.2.)

REQUIREMENTS AND ADVISABLE LIMITS

Lactose

While there is no evidence that lactose is an essential nutrient, we consider that its position as the mammalian milk sugar is a strong argument for a minimum lactose content in a formula, and that lactose should not be completely omitted unless symptoms of lactose intolerance make it necessary. There is little scientific evidence on which to base a minimum content, however. Since the use of formulas in LBW babies with a lactose content as low as 3.2 g per 100 kcal has been well documented (20) we accept this as empirical evidence of an acceptable lower limit. A further reduction below this lower limit should not be considered unless there is a clear need.

The upper limit for lactose content is related to intestinal tolerance. The amount tolerated by the intestine is probably more related to lactose concentration (*per dl*) and total intake (i.e. *per kg body weight per day*) rather than the content of lactose per 100 kcal. Despite the low concentrations of intestinal lactase found in the 30 week fetus, the enzyme presumably rises rapidly after birth since lactose intolerance is only an occasional problem in preterm babies receiving up to 200 ml/kg per day of either breast milk or many 'normal' formulas, i.e. lactose up to 7.8 g per dl, 15.6 g/kg per day, 11.7 g per 100 kcal. In one series, however, only 70% of LBW babies tolerated and thrived on a formula supplying 21.2 g/kg per day of lactose (10.6 g per dl; 13.2 g per 100 kcal). The remainder had frequent stools (21). Any upper limit might, therefore, be set somewhere between these two observations. In practice, however, a concentration greater than 7.8 g per dl or 11.7 g per 100 kcal (i.e. the amount in human milk) seems to have no particular advantages. There is no extensive experience of formulas with concentrations of lactose greater than 7.8 g per dl or 11.7 g per 100 kcal, and the limit allows sufficient flexibility for food technologists to control such facts as renal solute load, etc. This figure is rounded up to 8 g per dl and 12 g per 100 kcal.

Total carbohydrate

We are unaware of any extensive experience with formulas providing less carbohydrate than in whole cow's milk, i.e. 4.8 g per dl, 7.2 g per 100 kcal and we accept this, rounded down to 7 g per 100 kcal as the lower limit, i.e. a minimum of 26% of energy from carbohydrate, or if fed to provide 130 kcal per kg, 9.1 g per kg. Regarding the upper limit there are many formulas for normal and LBW babies containing up to 9.7 g per dl and 12.6 g per 100 kcal of carbohydrate (see Table 1.2) and experience with these has been satisfactory. Similarly an experimental formula containing total carbohydrate 10.6 g per dl, 13.3 g per 100 kcal, 5.6 g lactose, 7.6 sucrose, was satisfactory in all respects (21). A tentative upper limit of 11 g per dl (14 g per 100 kcal) is, therefore, suggested, i.e. a maximum of 56% energy from carbohydrate. We are concerned that this upper limit should not be interpreted too rigidly, however, and so curtailing further possible developments in infant formulas, for example a well absorbed carbohydrate might be an alternative to medium chain triglyceride as an energy source when long chain absorption was reduced. In these circumstances, with adequate trials, a total carbohydrate concentration greater than 11 g per dl or 14g per 100 kcal (i.e. 18.2 g/kg if fed to provide 130 kcal per kg) might be demonstrated as acceptable. We are aware that carbohydrate supplements may be added to breast milk to increase its energy content. This may well reduce the protein: energy ratio to levels well below that normally found in breast milk. This is undesirable.

Quality of carbohydrates

If other carbohydrates apart from lactose are used they must be 'acceptable' and acceptability can only be demonstrated by clinical investigation and trial. Small amounts of glucose may be acceptable but this increases osmolality and will eventually result in diarrhoea. The use of sucrose in infant formulas has been questioned but does not result in excessive deposition of fat nor in plasma lipid abnormalities in LBW babies, at least in the short term (21). It results in a greater secretion of insulin than does lactose (22). But this is not a clear disadvantage. We therefore consider that sucrose is an acceptable carbohydrate. Various starch hydrolysates are in widespread use; their constitution and osmolality vary according to the dextrose equivalent number and so each one must be shown clinically to be suitable (see Nutritional Background above). Although starch can be a source of energy (14) the low activity of pancreatic $\propto$-amylase (12), and the reduced weight gain in relation to energy intake seen in young infants (7) suggest that other carbohydrates are more suitable in the early weeks of life. We are not aware of galactose being used as an alternative carbohydrate source.

GUIDELINES

1 Only the occasional baby will be unable to tolerate the amount of lactose in breast milk and 'normal' formulas fed in volumes of up to 200 ml per kg per day, i.e. 7.8 g per dl, 11.7 g per 100 kcal, 15.6 g per kg. Carbohydrate supplements should not be added to breast milk to increase its energy content since this will reduce the protein:energy ratio.

2 In a formula:

(a) Lactose 3.2–12 g per 100 kcal and not more than 8 g per dl.

(b) Total carbohydrate 7–14 g per 100 kcal and not more than 11 g per 100 dl (a higher limit for total carbohydrate might be acceptable following suitable trials).

(c) Carbohydrates apart from lactose, which are acceptable are:

  (i) Glucose, so long as osmolality of the feed is not so excessive as to cause diarrhoea;

  (ii) starch hydrolysates, e.g. maltodextrins or corn syrup solids, which have been demonstrated by clinical investigation as acceptable;

  (iii) sucrose.

There are probably better alternatives to starch.

REFERENCES

1. Donnell G.N., Collado M. & Koch R. (1961). Growth and development of children with galactosemia. *J. Pediatr.* **58**, 836–44.
2. Vaughan O.W. & Filer L.J. Jr. (1960). The enhancing action of certain carbohydrates on the intestinal absorption of calcium in the rat. *J. Nutr.* **71**, 10–14.
3. Wasserman R.H. & Comar C.L. (1959). Carbohydrates and gastrointestinal absorption of radiostrontium and radiocalcium in the rat. *Proc. Soc. Exp. Biol. Med.* **101**, 314–17.
4. Armbrecht H.G. & Wasserman R.H. (1976). Enhancement of Ca^{++} uptake by lactose in the rate small intestine. *J. Nutr.* **106**, 1265–71.
5. Mills R., Breiter H., Kempster E., McKey B., Pickens M., & Outhouse J. (1940). The influence of lactose on calcium retention in children. *J. Nutr.* **20**, 467–76.
6. Kobayashi A., Kawai S., Ohbe Y. & Nagashima Y. (1975). Effects of dietary lactose and a lactase preparation on the intestinal absorption of calcium and magnesium in normal infants. *Am. J. Clin. Nutr.* **28**, 681–3.
7. Ziegler E.E. & Fomon S.J. (1982). Methods in infant nutrition research: balance and growth studies. *Acta Paediatr. Scand.* (Suppl.) **299**, 90–6.
8. Bullen C.L. & Willis A.T. (1971). Resistance of the breast-fed infant to gastroenteritis. *Br. Med. J.* **3**, 338–43.
9. Smallpiece V. & Davies P.A. (1964). Immediate feeding of premature infants with undiluted breast milk. *Lancet* **ii**, 1349–52.
10. Wharton B.A. & Bower B.D. (1965). Immediate or later feeding for premature babies: a controlled trial. *Lancet* **ii**, 969–72.
11. Auricchio S., Rubino A. & Murset G. (1965) Intestinal glycosidase activities in the human embryo, fetus and newborn. *Pediatrics* **35**, 944–54.

12. Zoppi G., Andreotti G., Pajno-Ferrara F., Njai D.M. & Gaburro D. (1972). Exocrine pancreas function in premature and full term neonates. *Pediatr. Res.* **6**, 880–2.
13. DeVizia B., Ciccimarra F., DeCicco N. & Auricchio S. (1975). Digestibility of starches in infants and children. *J. Pediatr.* **86**, 50–3.
14. Senterre J. (1980). Net absorption of starch in low birth weight infants. *Acta Paediatr. Scand.* **69**, 653–7.
15. Husband J., Husband P. & Mallinson C.N. Gastric emptying of starch meals in the newborn. *Lancet* ii, 290–2.
16. Anderson T.A., Fomon S.J. & Filer L.J. (1972). Carbohydrate tolerance with 3 day old infants. *J. Lab. Clin. Med.* **79**, 31–3.
17. Eggermont E. (1969). The hydrolysis of the naturally occuring α-glucosidases by the human intestinal mucosa. *Eur. J. Biochem.* **9**, 483.
18. Lebenthal E. & Lee R.D.C. (1980). Glucoamaylase and disaccharidase activities in normal subjects and in patients with mucosal injury of the small intestine. *J. Pediatr.* **97**, 389.
19. Cicco R., Holzman I.R., Brown D.R. & Becker D.J. (1981). Glucose polymer tolerance in premature infants. *Pediatrics* **67**, 498–501.
20. Jonxis J.H.P. (1976). Special problems arising in the nutrition of very small prematures and their subsequent growth. In: *Early Nutrition and Later Development* (ed. A.W. Wilkinson), pp 79–91.Pitman Medical, Kent.
21. Fosbrooke A.S. & Wharton B.A. (1975). Added lactose and added sucrose cows milk formulae in nutrition of low birth weight babies. *Arch Dis. Child.* **50**, 409–18.
22. Schmidt E. (1978). *Der Einflub verschiedener Kohlenhydrate in vergleich-baren Sauglings-mischnahrungen auf den Verlauf der Blutglukose-und Seruminsulinkurve.* Colloquium Deutschsprachiger Gastroenterologen, Hamburg.

7
Vitamins

Vitamins are a group of organic compounds which are essential in small amounts for specific metabolic functions; they cannot be synthesized in the body and must therefore be present in the diet.

Overt clinical signs of deficiency may occur only when severe and prolonged vitamin depletion has taken place, while minor deficiency states are often difficult to recognize on clinical grounds. Since the daily allowance of some vitamins will vary according to the amounts of other nutrients in the diet (1), and since toxicity is a rare event for most vitamins, the recommended intakes are generally calculated in excess of the true minimal requirements (1–13).

PLACENTAL TRANSFER

The vitamin endowment of the fetus at birth will to a certain extent influence the subsequent vitamin needs of the infant (10).

Lipid-soluble vitamins cross the placenta by simple and/or facilitated diffusion; their levels in fetal blood correlate well with the levels in maternal blood (14–16) being equal to or slightly lower than those in the mother, with the exception of vitamin E which is found in much lower concentration in cord blood (15,17). Their accumulation in fetal tissues takes place throughout pregnancy and is dependent on maternal blood levels. Blood concentrations at birth (14–16) and possibly body stores are lower than normal in preterm infants and in infants of poorly nourished mothers (18).

The levels of *water-soluble* vitamins are generally higher in fetal than in maternal blood (14,19). The presence of this concentration gradient suggests they cross the placenta by active transport (14), with the exception of vitamin C which crosses the placenta by facilitated diffusion in the oxidized form. Dehydro-ascorbic acid is then reduced by the fetus to ascorbic acid which crosses the placenta with difficulty and therefore accumulates on the fetal side (20).

AVAILABLE FOODS

There is a considerable variation in the concentration of vitamins in breast milk (15,16,19,21–26). This is probably due to differences in diet and nutritional status of the women studied, the season of the year, the prevailing weather, the stage of lactation and the methods used for assays (7,25,26,27).

Seasonal variations in vitamin levels have also been demonstrated in cow's milk, with higher values in the summer months (7,25–27). Vitamin levels in most of the commercially available formulae are generally equal to or higher than those found in human milk. However, the stability of some vitamins in the formula, both before and after reconstitution with water, is limited and a substantial reduction of the biological activity may occur with time, particularly following heat treatment, canning or light exposure (25,28).

On the other hand, it must be recognized that it is often difficult and sometimes impossible to correlate the vitamin content of available food with signs of deficiency in low birth weight (LBW) infants, since they are usually supplemented with various vitamin preparations in addition to the amounts introduced with feeds.

Where relevant, specific comments concerning the vitamin content of available food for LBW infants will be made when discussing each individual vitamin.

VITAMIN A

The active form of vitamin A is retinol, a fat soluble alcohol present as numerous isomers. Vitamin A can be derived from the transformation of various carotenoids, of which the most important is β carotene. Vitamin A activity is expressed as retinol equivalents (RE) or international units (iu).

1 RE=1 μg all-trans-retinol=3.33 iu Vitamin A=6 μg β carotene=12 μg
of other carotenoids (15).

Nutritional background

Vitamin A is transported in the plasma bound to a carrier protein, retinol binding protein (RBP), (29,30).

There is evidence in animals that the fetal liver does not synthesize RBP until quite late in gestation (31), and at least some of the RBP found in fetal plasma is of maternal origin, probably transported to the fetus in combination with retinol (32). Plasma concentrations of both retinol and RBP are lower in preterm than in term infants (33–39) and considerably lower than in maternal plasma (14,18,32,33). The molar ratio of retinol: RBP is also low in preterm infants (36), indicating increased amounts of unbound RBP in the plasma. It is not known whether this reflects a low rate of placental transfer or a rapid rate of utilization by the fetus. Deficiency of vitamin A in full term newborns has not been described.

Vitamin A in excess of requirement is stored in the liver and needs RBP for its mobilization. Vitamin A toxicity has only been described when very large amounts have been consumed for a long period of time (probably 500 μg for 6 weeks) and is characterized by vomiting and increased intracranial pressure (1,40).

The present information on the vitamin A status in VLBW infants is incomplete (15). The already mentioned low plasma levels of retinol in preterm infants (33–39) suggest that they have low body stores at birth and that they are at risk of developing a deficiency state (15). This is supported also by the recent finding of decreased vitamin A reserves in the liver of these neonates (41). Although a deficiency state has not been recognized clinically in VLBW babies, infants treated with prolonged ventilation for severe respiratory distress (42) and infants with bronchopulmonary dysplasia (43) have very low plasma concentrations of retinol, suggesting a subclinical deficiency state and/or an increased utilization of vitamin A.

Available foods

Human milk contains vitamin A mainly as retinol palmitate, in variable concentrations depending on the maternal diet (21,26,44).

Measured levels in pooled samples of mature milk range between 40 and 80 μg retinol/dl (average 60 μg/dl) and are about twice as high in colostrum (7,24). Vitamin A content of cow's milk is lower than that of human milk and is quite variable according to the season (higher in the summer) (7,27). Average retinol and carotene levels in cow's milk range between 27 and 36 μg/dl and between 12 and 21 μg/dl respectively (7). Proprietary formulas show variable levels of vitamin A (usually in the range of 50–100 μg/dl) depending on the origin of the fat and the amount added by the manufacturer

Requirements and advisable intakes

Precise requirements of vitamin A are unknown but 10 μg of retinol/kg body weight/day has been found to be sufficient for normally growing infants (45). An advisable intake of twice this amount (i.e 20 μg/kg per day) has therefore been proposed for young infants (1). Higher intakes (up to 480 μg/d) have been recommended by other official bodies during the first six months of life (5). In contrast with this recommendation vitamin A is often given in great excess of the estimated requirements. This is due to the fact that vitamin D and A are present together in the available vitamin preparations and when giving the appropriate dose of vitamin D the corresponding amount of vitamin A is excessive. On the other hand this practice has not produced apparent clinical toxicity in normal infants. Infants breast fed by well nourished mothers do not apparently get clinical vitamin A deficiency; therefore an allowance equivalent to the minimum intake of the fully breast-fed infant (60 μg/100 kcal) is likely to be adequate for normal infants (7). Vitamin A content of proprietary formulae should not fall below the average amount found in human milk (i.e 60 μg/dl) which is in line with previous recommendations (7). However, because of the low body stores at birth, the rapidly growing preterm infant may need more than this to ensure adequate tissue stores (15), but probably no more than recommended by Codex Alimentarius for full-term infants (150 μg/100 kcal) unless there is severe fat malabsorption. Therefore, we see no reason for a formula to contain more than 115 μg retinol/dl (~150 μg/100 kcal).

Summary of guidelines

Infants fed breast milk

Human milk appears to provide sufficient amounts of vitamin A for term infants but it is unknown if this is true for LBW infants as well. Although there is no firm evidence that LBW infants receiving breast milk require vitamin A supplementation, since studies of vitamin A status in unsupplemented infants have shown low retinol plasma levels, we support the current practice of supplementing these infants with vitamin A, from a minimum of 200 to a maximum of 1000 μg/d.

Artificially fed infants

Proprietary formulae for LBW infants, when reconstituted should contain vitamin A in a concentration not lower than that found in breast milk (90 μg/100 kcal) and not higher than the recommendation of Codex Alimentarius (150 μg/100 kcal).

VITAMIN D (CHOLECALCIFEROL)

Vitamin D activity is expressed in international units (iu): 1μg cholecalciferol = 40 iu vitamin D_3.

Nutritional background

Vitamin D_3 in plasma is bound to a specific binding protein (46); it is hydroxylated in the liver to 25 hydroxycholecalciferol (25-OH-D_3), which is the most abundant vitamin D_3 metabolite found in blood and in liver stores (47,48). Plasma levels of 25-OH-D_3 normally range between 8 and 55 μg/ml (49), and are useful indicators of the vitamin D status of the infant (47,50). Other metabolites, such as 24,25 and particularly the most active form 1,25-di-hydroxy-D_3 are present in much lower concentrations (1–6 μg/ml and 26–65 pg/ml respectively) in healthy adults (48,49).

The two naturally occurring forms of vitamin D, cholecalciferol and ergocalciferol, as well as other synthetic compounds such as 25-OH-D_3, $1\propto$-OH-D_3 and 1,25-$(OH)_2$-D_3 are all biologically active when administered to babies (47,48).

Fetal endowment of vitamin D depends on maternal vitamin D blood levels during pregnancy, which in turn are related to maternal vitamin D nutrition and sunlight exposure (51,52). At birth preterm infants have plasma 25-OH-vitamin D levels which are related to maternal levels but are generally lower than those found in their mothers (51–61), possibly because of the low concentration of vitamin D binding protein (58). Congenital rickets may occur in neonates from mothers with vitamin D deficiency (16,59,61,62); however, rickets usually occurs beyond the neonatal period, after vitamin D deficiency has been present for some time. Lack of vitamin D, particularly when body stores at birth are low and when cow's milk is fed, can also cause neonatal tetany due to hypocalcaemia (16,50,59,62). Relative vitamin D deficiency has been implicated in the pathogenesis of poor bone mineralization which has been frequently described in preterm infants, particularly in those of very low gestational age (16,51,59,61,62). Relative fat malabsorption and insufficient bile salt production in LBW infants may contribute to vitamin D deficiency (16,51).

However, the pathogenesis of these skeletal lesions is most often multifactorial and the role of vitamin D in each individual case needs to be established (16,51) (see section on calcium). In infants of more than 32 weeks gestation with low 25-OH-D_3 plasma concentration at birth, provision of 20–50 μg vitamin D_3 per day results in increased plasma 25-OH-D_3 and 1,25-$(OH)_2$-D_3 within the first five days of administration, suggesting that these infants can absorb and hydroxylate vitamin D, provided the parent substrate is given in adequate amounts (63–69). Lower doses may be sufficient at later ages (65,68).

The feed-back regulation of 1,25-$(OH)_2$-D_3 synthesis also appears to be operative since low intakes of calcium and phosphorus as well as the administration of vitamin D or 25-OH-D_3 will produce higher levels of the metabolite in plasma (16,64,67,69).

Finally, the gut of preterm infants of more than 32 weeks gestation has been shown to respond to a pharmacological dose of $1,25\text{-}(OH)_2\text{-}D_3$ (0.5 μg) with a significant increase in calcium absorption (70–72). However, these mechanisms may not be fully operative in preterm infants of less than 32 weeks gestational age (50,51,73–75). Indeed, in 12 infants averaging less than 32 weeks of gestation, Cifuentes *et al.* found that seven had plasma $25\text{-}OH\text{-}D_3$ levels below the normal adult range (less than 8 μg/ml) when receiving 500 iu vitamin D /kg per day for up to three weeks (76). However, over a longer period (three months) vitamin D_3 intakes of 800 iu per day, in combination with a standard formula, resulted in good bone mineralization and elevation of plasma levels of $25\text{-}OH\text{-}D_3$ (76). Furthermore, in preterm infants fed human milk or formula, vitamin D supplementation (1200 iu day) has been shown to improve calcium absorption significantly (71,72). Vitamin D toxicity is usually iatrogenic, and it is characterized by pallor, nausea, vomiting, failure to thrive, polyuria, hypercalciuria, hypercalcemia and ectopic calcifications (1). Usually these signs will be produced by large amounts of vitamin D, more than 250 μg/kg per day, but cases have been described with prolonged intakes in the range of 100 μg per day (1,16).

Available foods

Breast-fed term infants rarely develop rickets and this has been taken as evidence that human milk usually contains sufficient amounts of vitamin D to meet the requirements of normal growing infants (77). However, there is still uncertainty concerning the vitamin D content of human milk and the nature of the biologically active metabolites present in it. Measurements by various authors (16,26,78) have yielded values between 0.1 and 0.2 μg/dl of cholecalciferol, contained in the lipid fraction.

Some authors have reported the presence of a water-soluble sulphate of vitamin D in human milk (79,80). However, more recently other authors, using more sophisticated analytical techniques, have failed to confirm these findings (26,81). Furthermore, specifically synthesized vitamin D sulphate has been found to have only 1–5% of the biological activity of vitamin D (16,26,81).

The most recent available evidence, based on measurements obtained with high performance liquid chromatography and radio-binding assay techniques, indicates that the total biological antirachitic steroid activity of breast milk is probably in the range of 1–8 iu/dl (0.03–0.2 μg/dl), depending on the maternal vitamin D status and the season of the year, and is largely due to $25\text{-}OH\text{-}D_3$ (16,26).

The concentration of vitamin D in cow's milk is even lower than in human milk; approximately 0.02 μg/dl (16).

Proprietary formulae contain variable amounts of vitamin D depending on the addition by the manufacturers, usually between 1 and 2 μg/dl.

Requirements and advisable intakes

It is recommended that full term growing infants should receive 10 μg (400 iu) of vitamin D/day (1,77). This recommended allowance is certainly in excess of the minimal requirements which is probably not higher than 2.5 μg (100 iu/d) (1). However, several studies suggest that preterm infants have higher requirements of vitamin D than full term infants, in the range of 800–1600 iu/day (20 to 40 μg/day), not only because their velocity of growth is greater, but because their vitamin D stores at birth will be less and the biotransformation pathways of vitamin D, though operational, may not be fully developed, particularly below 32 weeks gestational age (50,51,72,73,75,76,82). Also, the intestinal absorption of vitamin D may be limited due to a deficiency in bile salt production and fat absorption (51). More efficient absorption of hydroxylated vitamin D derivatives is possible, since this occurs in the upper small intestine and does not have as great a requirement for bile salts (51). The administration of 25-OH-D$_3$ during the first days of life at a dose of 2–10 μg/day has been shown to increase rapidly the 25-OH-D$_3$ plasma levels (63,74). However, its administration at higher doses and for longer periods of time may be dangerous since it can lead to accumulation and toxicity due to the long half-life of this compound (50,74,82).

The use of $1\propto$-OH-D$_3$ and even more that of 1.25-(OH)$_2$-D$_3$ should be considered experimental at present since the experience with these compounds is still limited, and since they can rapidly lead to toxicity though they are rapidly eliminated (10). Their use should, therefore, be limited to those cases where plasma levels of the various vitamin D metabolites and calcium can be monitored.

Summary of guidelines

All infants

The vitamin D requirements of LBW infants are influenced by the body stores at birth, which in turn are related to the length of gestation, the maternal diet and maternal exposure to sunlight. These factors should be taken into consideration when deciding the policy concerning vitamin D supplementation in each institution. Vitamin D (chole- or ergo-calciferol) is preferred for supplementation; other metabolites and alphacalcidol should be used only in special circumstances. The supplementation suggested here should be stopped when the baby is discharged from the hospital or reaches term: thereafter vitamin D supplement should be the same as in term infants (400 iu/day).

Infants fed human milk

When human milk is used, LBW infants should be supplemented on the average with 1000 iu (25 μg/day) of vitamin D $_3$; supplementation should not be less than 800 iu/day and not more than 1600 iu/day.

Artificially fed infants

Because of individual variations in the sensitivity to vitamin D it would be unwise for all of this to be provided by a formula. Therefore, the vitamin D content of proprietary formulae for LBW infants should not exceed 3 μg (120 iu)/100 kcal. Vitamin D should be in the form of chole-or ergo-calciferol.

Artificially fed LBW infants should be supplemented with vitamin D in order to achieve a total intake of 1000 iu/day (including the amount given with feeds), and not less than 800 or more than 1600 iu/day.

VITAMIN E

Vitamin E activity is expressed both as tocopherol equivalents (TE) and international units (iu)

1 iu = 1 TE = 1 mg dl - $\propto$-tocopherol-acetate = 0.97 mg/dl-$\propto$-tocopherol = 0.73 mg d $\propto$-tocopherol.

Nutritional background

Vitamin E is a powerful antioxidant and it protects polyunsaturated lipids of cell membranes from oxidation (83). Vitamin E also plays a role in the synthesis of haem for haemoglobin, cytochromes and other haem proteins and in the incorporation of iron into protopophirin IX. Iron administration may increase the need for vitamin E, since it catalyses the oxidation of cell lipids, through the generation of free radicals, and interferes with vitamin E absorption by increasing its destruction in the gut (15,84,85). Furthermore, since the lipid composition of cell membranes reflects the composition of dietary fats, the daily need for vitamin E is related to the amount of polyunsaturated fatty acid (PUFA) in the diet. Experiments in animals and in man (86–88), as well as clinical experience, have indicated that a supply of 0.6 mg of d-$\propto$-tocopherol per 1 g of PUFA is sufficient to prevent lipid peroxidation and other signs of vitamin E deficiency, such as increased platelet function and enhanced oxidative hemolysis of red cells *in vitro* (89,90). Clinical signs of deficiency are rare but haemolytic anaemia and peripheral oedema have been described in preterm infants fed diets with low $\propto$-tocopherol/PUFA ratios (91–93). Plasma concentrations of vitamin E at birth are low, particularly in preterm infants, due to limited passage of this vitamin and possibly total lipids across the placenta (14,15,17,18,94–98). Deficiency states are associated with low plasma levels of $\propto$-tocopherol (below 0.5mg/dl) (99). However, these levels have little meaning if not related to plasma lipid concentrations (100). A plasma ratio of $\propto$-tocopherol to total lipids above 0.5, as suggested by Horwitt *et al.* (100), should be considered normal (101). Another indicator of vitamin E status could be the tocopherol concentration in cell membranes, such as for example, in the red cells (102). Decreased osmotic resistance of red cells to oxidative agents *in vitro* is a reliable test of vitamin E deficiency (103) and correlates well with very low plasma vitamin E concentrations and with low tocopherol/lipid ratios in preterm infants (92,104,105).

Increased intakes and sometimes pharmacological doses of vitamin E have been proposed for the prevention and/or treatment of a variety of clinical conditions peculiar to the preterm infant, such as bronchopulmonary dysplasia (BPD), retinopathy of prematurity (ROP), intraventricular haemorrhage (IVH) and anaemia of prematurity (106,107). Although retinopathy of prematurity cannot be regarded as a vitamin E deficiency disease, vitamin E may be protective in vulnerable infants (107–109), since there is evidence that large supplements given from the first day of life diminish both the incidence and severity of ROP and treatment of infants with established disease has resulted in improvement (107–115). An initial report (116) that vitamin E supplementation reduces the incidence of bronchopulmonary dysplasia has not been confirmed (117–122). Preterm infants given vitamin E supplements have been observed to have a lower incidence of intraventricular haemorrhage than non-supplemented infants (123–125), but the mechanism is obscure and the results have been challenged and need to be confirmed by other studies (126, 127).

There is also much controversy concerning the need of supplementing the diet of LBW infants with vitamin E for the prevention of anaemia of prematurity (15,90). Most of the studies suggesting a beneficial effect of such a supplementation have been performed without proper randomization of cases and controls, or in infants fed formulae with inadequate tocopherol/PUFA ratios (90). Furthermore, the reported beneficial effects on haemoglobin levels have often been small (less than 0.6 g/dl on the average) and therefore of limited clinical significance (84,90,92,104,128–131). Finally, other studies have failed to show any clinical benefit from such a supplementation (90,91,104,132–136).

Toxicity from vitamin E has been mostly studied in animals and results in inhibition of prostaglandin synthesis in platelets, decreased platelet aggregation, increased haemorrhagic tendency in vitamin K deficiency, decreased fibrinolytic activity and creatinuria (90).

Overt signs of toxicity due to high vitamin E intakes have not been described in adults with doses as high as 800 μg/day (137). Initial reports in preterm infants have also denied clear signs of toxicity even with pharmacological doses (30–100 mg/kg per day) of vitamin E (15,90,109,138). However, more recently, a possible association between prolonged high serum levels of vitamin E ($>$5 mg/dl) and sepsis and necrotizing entercolitis has been suggested in preterm infants (139). Therefore, it has been recommended that when vitamin E is administered in pharmacological doses (25–100 mg/kg per day) to LBW infants, plasma levels should be monitored and maintained within the normal adult range (below 4 mg/dl) (140). This seems logical since plasma levels above 1 mg/dl are usually associated with adequate tissue stores (102,141). The type of preparation used and the route of administration are also important (142) since hyperosmolar solutions may damage the intestinal mucosa (143), intravenous administration may produce dangerously high plasma levels (140) and the i.v. injection of tocopherol acetate has been associated with severe toxicity and death in preterm infants (140,144,145).

Available foods

Human milk content of $\propto$-tocopherol ranges between 0.29 and 0.54 mg TE/dl (average 0.40) (7,90). The average ratio between $\propto$-tocopherol (mg) and PUFA (mainly linoleic acid) (g) in human milk is around 0.7–1.1 and in any case it is always higher than 0.4 (5,90). Cow's milk content of $\propto$-tocopherol is lower (average 0.09 mg/dl) and shows seasonal variations as with other fat soluble vitamins (5,27). The ratio $\propto$-tocopherol/PUFA (linoleic acid) is also substantially lower in cow's milk than in breast milk (0.4 vs 0.8) (7).

Proprietary formulae complying with recent recommendations contain variable amounts of vitamin E (0.3–2.2 mg/dl), depending on the total amount of PUFA present and an $\propto$-tocopherol/PUFA ration always higher than 0.4 (9).

Requirements and advisable intakes

Since the requirements of vitamin E are related to the quality and quantity of fats in the diet and since intestinal absorption is incomplete and variable it is practically impossible to define the absolute minimal requirements (15). However, breast-fed full term infants do not show signs of vitamin E deficiency and therefore the amount of $\propto$-tocopherol in human milk appears adequate for them. Although a ratio of $\propto$-tocopherol (mg/PUFA) (g) of 0.4 has been reported as safe, a higher ratio (0.7/1, i.e. the same as in breast milk) has been recommended in premature infants (3,6,7,12,90). The claim of some authors

(146) that oral vitamin E is poorly absorbed in LBW infants has not been confirmed by others (147–150), though the intestinal absorption and bioavailability of vitamin E in preterm infants fed human milk, and particularly preterm milk, seems to be better than in infants receiving artificial formula (85). Therefore, we recommend that both the absolute amount of vitamin E as well as the ratio between vitamin E and PUFA (linoleic acid) in proprietary formulae for LBW infants should not be lower than the average values found in human milk (i.e. 0.40 mg TE/dl and 0.9 mg/1 g of PUFA).

Although the data presently available in the literature are somewhat contradictory and do not provide conclusive evidence for the need to supplement the diet of LBW infants with vitamin E, a recent report has indicated that the administration of iron (2 mg/kg per day) may indeed increase the need for vitamin E and some infants, particularly those fed proprietary formulae, may show biochemical evidence of vitamin E deficiency at six weeks of age (85). The oral administration of 4.1 mg/d of vitamin E after the first week of life was sufficient to prevent these abnormalities and was associated with normal haematological findings (85). Therefore, if it is elected to supplement LBW infants with vitamin E, a daily oral allowance of 5 mg is adequate and safe and it is in line with previous recommendations as well as with the common practice in many centres (3,12,15,85).

From the available data we cannot define an upper limit of vitamin E intake in LBW infants. However, because of the concern expressed on the possible toxicity of abnormally high plasma levels in LBW infants, we do not recommend prolonged (more than 1 week) oral administration of more than 50 mg of vitamin E/day (25 mg/day i.m.) in preterm infants. In any case plasma levels should be measured and the dosage adjusted accordingly.

For the same reason and since most European centres appear to have lower incidences of ROP than have been reported in vitamin E supplementation trials in the USA, we, as others (151), do not feel justified in recommending the routine administration of large doses of vitamin E to all preterm infants at present, but if it is elected to follow such a policy, a single oral dose of 50 mg on the first day of life (25 mg i.m.), followed by a daily oral administration of 5–7 mg/day has been shown to afford vitamin E plasma levels in the range of those described as 'protective' (102).

Summary of guidelines

Infants fed breast milk

Human milk provides sufficient amounts of vitamin E and an adequate α-tocopherol/PUFA ratio for LBW infants, and there is no conclusive evidence that supplementation is needed.

Artificially fed infants

The vitamin E content of formulae for LBW infants should not fall below 0.4 mg of TE/dl of reconstituted formula (0.6 mg/100 kcal) and should guarantee an α-tocopherol/PUFA ratio of at least 0.9 mg/g.

Prevention of anaemia

The difference in haemoglobin concentration following routine supplementation with vitamin E (5–20 mg/day) is in our opinion not sufficiently large for us to recommend that such supplementation is essential in breast-fed infants or in infants fed formulae complying with Recommendation No. 2. However, if such a policy is followed, an oral supplement of 5 mg/day is both adequate and safe.

VITAMIN K

Nutritional background

Vitamin K is necessary for the hepatic synthesis of active prothrombin and coagulation factors VII, IX and X. Therefore, deficiency of vitamin K is accompanied by low plasma levels of the above mentioned coagulation proteins, prolongation of the coagulation time and prothrombin time, and bleeding tendency (15,152,153).

Vitamin K is needed in very small amounts (less than 0.5 μg/kg per day) (15). However, since its intestinal absorption may range between 40 and 70%, a daily allowance of 1 μg/kg per day has been suggested in adults (5,15). Vitamin K is also synthesized by the microbiological flora in the gut and roughly 50% of the total intake may be derived by this source (15). A deficiency state is very seldom observed except in the neonate. It can occur when lack of dietary intake or absorption is associated with prolonged antibiotic treatment (15,154,155). In those instances, however, deficiency can occur very rapidly since body stores are limited and the turnover is very fast (156). Circulating vitamin K levels are low (0.2–8 ng/ml) (157,158) and difficult to measure, therefore the adequacy of vitamin K status is usually assessed by the prothrombin time assay (15). By this method as well as by direct measurements it has been shown that plasma levels are low at birth, particularly in preterm infants (158–161), suggesting a limited transfer of vitamin K across the placenta (15). Indeed, it is well known that newborn infants and particularly LBW infants, can develop a bleeding tendency (haemorrhagic disease of the newborn) due to the limited stores at birth, to the lack of synthesis in the gut (not colonized as yet) and to the small amounts supplied with milk, particularly breast milk (1,15,152).

Recently attention has been drawn to the occurrence of vitamin K deficiency beyond the neonatal period, in exclusively breast-fed infants (162–166). Very low levels of vitamin K in their mother's breast milk, lack of administration of vitamin K at birth, poor absorption, antibiotic treatment, have all been implicated in this form of 'late haemorrhagic disease', which is particularly severe since it is often associated with intracranial bleeding (165,166). Vitamin K toxicity in the form of haemolytic anaemia and jaundice has been observed in newborn infants following the administration of synthetic vitamin K analogues (menadione) which are not used any more (1,167).

Available foods

Human milk contains very small amounts of vitamin K: between 1 and 2 μg/dl (7,15,24,152,168). Cow's milk content of vitamin K is higher, ranging between 1 and 8.5 μg/dl (average 6 μg/dl) (7,15,152,153,168,169).

Proprietary formulae usually contain more vitamin K than human milk (3–10 μg/dl) (168,169).

Requirements and advisable intakes

Daily dietary requirements of vitamin K have not been determined with certainty due to the variable amounts that are synthesized and absorbed in the gut (1,15). They must, however, be quite low, probably in the range of 0.1–0.5 μg/kg per day, since bleeding due to vitamin K deficiency is rare, except during the first ten days of life when milk intake is still insufficient. For this reason it has been recommended that all infants should receive 0.5–1 mg of vitamin K on the first day of life (7,15,154,155,166). Although vitamin K is well asborbed from the gut (170), it is probably best to give it intramuscularly in VLBW infants to ensure an early and adequate effect. In infants who are exclusively fed with human milk, or when oral feeding is delayed, or when antibiotics are used, this dose should be repeated at weekly intervals or, alternatively, a daily allowance of 2 μg/kg per day should be provided (15,166).

Summary of guidelines

All LBW infants should receive 0.5–1 mg of vitamin K, preferably i.m., on the first day of life. This dose should be repeated at weekly intervals until adequate feeding is instituted.

Infants fed breast milk

An oral daily allowance of 2–3 μg/kg of vitamin K is suggested after the first week of life.

Artificially fed infants

Proprietary formulae for LBW infants should contain at least 4 μg of vitamin K per 100 kcal. Although an upper limit cannot be indicated with certainty, we see no reason to exceed 15 μg/100 kcal.

THIAMIN (VITAMIN B$_1$)

Nutritional background

Thiamine is transformed by the liver into its active phosphorylated metabolite thiamin pyrophosphate or cocarboxylase, a coenzyme essential for carbohydrate metabolism. Overt signs of deficiency (beri-beri) are extremely rare in the newborn period. They can occur in infants fed non-supplemented soy milk, in infants breast-fed by alcoholic mothers with thiamin deficiency, in infants breast-fed by vitamin B$_1$ deficient mothers from underdeveloped countries or during unsupplemented parenteral nutrition (1). Since thiamin is readily excreted in urine toxicity from overdosage does not occur (1,19).

Available foods

Both human and cow's milk contain substantial amounts of thiamine and thiamine pyrophosphate. In fresh breast milk these two compounds behave differently during lactation. Thiamine remains roughly constant, between 10 and 13 μg/dl, while thiamine pyrophosphate increases rapidly from 0.1 to 9.4 μg/dl during the first 4 weeks post-partum and more slowly (up to 16.4 μg/dl) during the following two months (24,171,172).

Fresh cow's milk contains twice as much thiamine and thiamine pyrophosphate as mature human milk (1,172).

Proprietary formulae are usually supplemented with thiamine in concentrations ranging between 40 and 200 μg/dl (19). However, since thiamine is inactivated by heat the amounts present in the milk given to the baby (both breast milk and formula) may vary with the method used for the preparation of the feed and may be lower than expected (28).

Requirements and advisable intakes

Requirements of thiamine are related to energy intake and particularly to carbohydrate intake and have been estimated at around 20 μg/100 kcal per day (1,173).

Infants fed breast milk usually receive at least the estimated requirement and excess thiamine is eliminated in urine (1,171). On the other hand thiamine deficiency does not occur in breast-fed infants of normal mothers and therefore the amounts present in human milk seem sufficient (1). Since thiamine is inactivated by heat the above mentioned findings may not apply when heat treated human milk is used for feeding (28). When proprietary formulae are used their thiamin content should not be lower than 20 μg/100 kcal (15 μg/dl reconstituted feed).

Summary of guidelines

Infants fed breast milk

There is no evidence that thiamin supplementation is needed in LBW infants fed fresh or frozen and thawed breast milk. However, since thiamin is heat labile, supplementation is needed when heat-treated human milk is fed in order to guarantee a thiamin intake of at least 20 μg/100 kcal (25 μg/kg per day).

Artificially fed infants

Proprietary formulae for LBW infants should contain, at least 20 μg/100 kcal of thiamin when reconstituted. An upper limit cannot be set; however formulae with up to 250 μg/100 kcal have been fed to preterm infants without apparent harm.

RIBOFLAVIN (VITAMIN B$_2$)

Nutritional background

There is little information on vitamin B$_2$ metabolism in the newborn. However, neither frank riboflavin deficiency nor toxicity have been described in term newborn infants. Laboratory diagnosis of riboflavin deficiency is based on the activation of red-cell glutathion-reductase by FAD *in vitro*; an activation coefficient of 1.2 or higher is strongly suggestive of a deficiency state (1).

Available foods

Human milk contains about 30–50 μg of riboflavin/dl (40–70 μg/100 kcal) (24,25). Cow's milk content is higher, ranging between 150 and 230 μg/dl (average 190 μg/dl) (25). Most proprietary formulae have higher contents than human milk, in the range of 60–300 μg/dl.

Requirements and advisable intakes

The need for riboflavin is related to energy metabolism: a daily allowance of 40–60 μg/100 kcal has been shown to be adequate (174).

Normal breast-fed infants don't show signs of deficiency, hence the riboflavin content of human milk must be adequate.

However, since riboflavin is subject to photodegradation its concentration may decrease in human milk exposed to light for variable periods of time (175). Futhermore it has been suggested that phototherapy may cause a transient riboflavin deficiency in breast-fed infants (175,176). Finally, a recent report has provided evidence of transient riboflavin depletion in preterm infants fed exclusively human milk; however, no clinical signs of deficiency were observed (175). Proprietary formulae should contain at least the amount present in human milk. An upper limit cannot be set, though proprietary formulae with up to 600 μg of riboflavin/100 kcal have been used without apparent untoward effects.

Summary of recommendations

Infants fed breast milk

The daily intake of riboflavin in breast-fed infants is 60 μg/100 kcal and there is no firm evidence that supplementation is needed.

Artificially fed infants

Proprietary formulae for LBW infants should contain at least as much riboflavin as human milk (i.e. 40 μg/dl; 60 μg/100 kcal). An upper limit cannot be set but we see no reason for exceeding what is present in available formulas (i.e. 600 μg/100 kcal).

NICOTINIC ACID (NIACIN, VITAMIN B₃, VITAMIN PP)

Nutritional background

In man niacin can also be synthesized from tryptophane in the presence of pyridoxine (vitamin B_6), when the aminoacid exceeds minimal requirements in the diet: 60 mg of tryptophane yield 1 mg of niacin (1). Thus the niacin content of food is best expressed by the 'niacin equivalent', which includes both niacin as such and the amount of niacin that can be generated by the tryptophane in excess of minimal requirements:

1 niacin equivalent (NE) = niacin (mg) + (tryptophane (mg) x 0.017)

Niacin deficiency causes pellagra which is characterized by dermatitis, diarrhoea and neurological symptoms. However, frank pellagra usually results from multiple vitamin deficiencies and insufficient protein intakes.

Neither niacin deficiency not toxicity have been observed in newborn infants.

Available foods

Human milk contains approximately 230 μg/dl of niacin and cow's milk approximately 100 μg/dl (24). However, approximately 70% of the niacin equivalents (NE) in breast milk, and 90% in cow's milk are contributed by tryptophan (19). Therefore, breast milk provides approximately 0.6 NE/dl (0.85 NE/100 kcal) and cow's milk about 1 NE/dl. Most proprietary formulae contain higher amounts in the range of 500–1000 μg/dl (7,19) of niacin, with a variable tryptophan content.

Requirements and advisable intakes

The need for niacin is related to energy intake and it has been recommended not to fall below 400 μg/100 kcal ($\sim$500 μg/kg per day) (1). However, since niacin can be synthesized from tryptophan the requirement should be expressed as NE and should not fall below 0.8 NE/100 kcal (5).

Human milk has been shown to provide enough niacin to prevent deficiency. Proprietary formulae should, therefore, have a content of niacin (or NE) at least equal to that of human milk.

An upper limit cannot be set, although artificial formulae with up to 5 NE/100 kcal have been used without apparent harm.

Summary of guidelines

Infants fed breast milk

The niacin content of human milk seems to be adequate and there is no evidence that supplementation is needed in LBW infants fed human milk.

Artificially fed infants

Proprietary formulae for LBW infants should contain at least 800 μg/100 kcal of niacin (or 0.8 NE). An upper limit cannot be set but we see no reason to exceed what is present in available formulae (i.e. 5 NE/100 kcal).

PANTOTHENIC ACID (VITAMIN B$_5$)

Nutritional background

Isolated deficiency of pantothenic acid has only been produced experimentally, but never described clinically, since the diet always provides sufficient amounts (19).

Available foods

Human milk contains about 250 μg of pantothenic acid per dl and cow's milk 350 μg/dl. Most proprietary formulae have higher amounts (200–400 μg/dl) (7,19,24).

Requirements and advisable intakes

Minimal requirements of pantothenic acid are unknown. Breast milk and proprietary formulae provide sufficient amounts for the young infant.

Summary of recommendations

Infants fed breast milk

There is no evidence that LBW infants fed human milk need to be supplemented with pantothenic acid.

Artificially fed infants

Formulae for LBW infants should contain at least 200 μg of pantothenic acid/dl reconstituted feed (330 μg/100 kcal). An upper limit cannot be set.

PYRIDOXIN (VITAMIN B$_6$)

Various compounds such as pyridoxin, pyridoxal and pyridoxamine all show vitamin B$_6$ activity. Vitamin B$_6$ is heat stable but is inactivated by light.

Nutritional background

Dietary deficiency of vitamin B_6 has been described in infants (177); it is accompanied by vomiting, irritability, dermatitis, failure to thrive, anaemia and finally convulsions (probably related to decreased synthesis of $\propto$-aminobutyric acid in the developing brain). Drugs, such as isoniazide and penicillamine, compete with or inactivate pyridoxine and may therefore increase its need or produce deficiency (1). Toxicity has never been reported in infants.

Available foods

The vitamin B_6 concentration (i.e. the sum of pyridoxine, pyridoxal and pyridoxamine) in human milk changes during lactation (24,178), from 47 μg/dl during the first 2–3 post-partum days to 23 μg/dl after one month. Cow's milk has a higher content (about 40 μg/dl) and so do most proprietary formulae (40–200 μg/dl) (7).

Requirements and advisable intakes

Requirements of vitamin B_6 are related to protein intake; it has been recommended that 15 μg of pyridoxin should be available per g of protein in the diet (1). Minimum requirements in LBW infants will thus vary according to the amount of protein in the diet. A daily allowance as high as 300 μg/day has been recommended for young infants, on the basis of the excretion of vitamin B_6 metabolites in urine (178). On the other hand the urinary excretion of $\propto$-pyridoxic acid during breast feeding is remarkably constant at 35 μg/day, and vitamin B_6 in breast-fed infants seems to be better retained in the body than in formula fed infants (178).

Furthermore, deficiency states have not been described in breast-fed infants; thus human milk seems to provide sufficient amounts of vitamin B_6 for the normal growing infant (1,19). Proprietary formulae should contain at least as much vitamin B_6 as human milk (25 μg/dl, 35 μg/100 kcal) and in any case not less than 15 μg/g protein.

This, however, may not be sufficient for LBW infants who are growing more rapidly and for whom a daily allowance of 60 μg/100 kcal has been recommended (3,19).

Summary of guidelines

Infants fed breast milk

LBW infants fed human milk may need to be supplemented with vitamin B_6 in order to achieve an intake of at least 15 μg/g protein and/or 35 μg/100 kcal.

Artificially fed infants

Proprietary formulae for LBW infants should contain at least 15 μg of vitamin B_6 per g of protein and not less than 25 μg/dl of reconstituted feed (35 μg/100 kcal). An upper limit cannot be set. However, we see no reason to exceed what is present in available formulae (250 μg/100 kcal).

BIOTIN (VITAMIN B_8)

Nutritional background

Deficiency states in man have been produced only experimentally by the administration of great amounts of an anti-vitamin, avidine, present in the egg-white. Clinical signs include pallor, anaemia, dermatitis, muscle-pain, lethargy and EEG abnormalities (174,179). Biotin deficiency syndromes have been found in inherited metabolic disorders of biotin conversion to its active metabolite, with the symptoms of severe muscle hypotonia, alopecia, acidosis, erythematous skin changes, propionic acidemia, and urinary excretion of methylcitrate, β-methyl-crotonylglycine and β-hyroxyisovalerate (180,181).

Biotin deficiency has also been observed with total parenteral nutrition (182,183). Since biotin is also synthesized by the intestinal flora and well absorbed in the gut, dietary deficiency is difficult to produce and daily requirements cannot be determined (1). Toxicity from biotin has not been reported.

Available foods

Human milk contains about 0.8 μg/dl of biotin; higher amounts are present in cow's milk (2 μg/dl) and in most proprietary formulae (1–3 μg/dl) (7,24).

Requirements and advisable intakes

Since biotin is synthesized in the gut (and well absorbed) minimal dietary requirements cannot be estimated with certainty. Breast-fed infants don't show signs of deficiency and hence the usual amount provided by breast feeding (approximately 1.2 μg/kg per day) must be sufficient (7,24). Proprietary formulae should therefore contain at least the amount present in human milk.

Summary of guidelines

Infants fed breast milk

There is no evidence that LBW infants fed human milk need to be supplemented with biotin.

Artificially fed infants

The biotin content of proprietary formulae for LBW infants should not fall below 1 μg/dl of reconstituted feed (1.5 μg/100 kcal). An upper limit cannot be set.

FOLIC ACID

Folic acid is destroyed by heat and canning and is inactivated by light.

Nutritional background

Lack of folic acid causes megaloblastic anaemia in infants, associated with leucopenia, thrombocytopenia, growth retardation, mucosal lesions in the small intestine and delayed CNS maturation (1,184,185,186).

Deficiency states can occur not only because of insufficient supply in the diet, but more commonly because of poor absorption due to malabsorption syndromes (187). Some drugs such as phenobarbitone and phenytoin increase the need for folic acid, probably through the induction of hepatic enzymes containing folic acid as a coenzyme (1,188). Requirements for folic acid are increased in pregnancy, during intense haemopoiesis and during growth (185,189–191).

The limited body reserves at birth together with the rapid post-natal growth and cell division probably increase the need for folic acid in LBW infants (184,189–191). Megaloblastic anaemia as a consequence of folic acid deficiency has been described in LBW infants (192–194). On the other hand, anaemia is a late sign of folic acid deficiency (195) and other more subtle morphological changes in erythrocytes and leucocytes, often described in LBW infants, have been interpreted as more sensitive indicators of subclinical deficiency states (184,194,196).

The clinical results of folic acid supplementation in LBW infants are also somewhat controversial, in that a clear haematological response has not always followed(197–201). However, it has been shown that a test dose of folic acid given to newborn infants disappears from the blood more rapidly than in older subjects, without any increase in the amount excreted in the urine (190), and this has been interpreted as evidence for an increased need of this vitamin.

Another explanation for this finding is also possible. Kamen & Caston (202) and Fernandes-Costa & Metz (203) have demonstrated high concentrations of a folate binding protein in human umbilical cord serum, different from that found in serum from pregnant women. The apparently increased disappearance of a test dose may thus be due to the increased binding to this protein and not to increased utilization. Toxicity from folic acid has never been described in infancy (184). Intakes of 155 μg/day for 3 months in preterm infants have not produced untoward effects.

Available foods

Human and cow's milk have a low content of folic acid (7,24,204,205). However, folic acid levels in breast milk increase rapidly after the first post-partum week, from 0.5–1 μg/dl to 2–4 μg at one month and up to 5–10 μg/dl at 3 months (206,107).

Also, folic acid in human milk seems to be better absorbed and utilized than in cow's milk or formula. It is likely that with improved chemical methods for analysis higher values will be found than previously reported (208). Proprietary formulae show a wide range of folic acid concentrations, from undetectable levels to 15 μg/dl.

Requirements and advisable intakes

Normal breast-fed infants do not show signs of folic acid deficiency and their plasma and red cell folate concentration as well as tissue saturation must be considered to be normal (1,184,209,210).

Therefore, fresh human milk provides sufficient folic acid under normal circumstances. This corresponds to a daily intake of 5–10 μg/kg which is what is usually recommended. As already mentioned, however, LBW infants may show subclinical evidence of folic acid deficiency with such intakes. In these infants 60–65 μg/day of folic acid has been shown to correct serum folic acid levels and erythrocyte and leucocyte morphology (184,189,209,210).

Since the danger of toxicity is non-existent, it seems advisable to provide this intake in LBW infants. Proprietary formulae for LBW infants should preferably contain sufficient folic acid to provide an intake of 60 μg/day even in the smallest infants (about 40 μg/dl). This may be impossible due to the rapid inactivation of folic acid following heat treatment, canning and exposure to light. Therefore, it seems advisable to supplement LBW infants with folic acid to guarantee that minimal requirements are met (184).

Summary of guidelines

Infants fed breast milk

Human milk, particularly after heat-treatment and storage, may not provide sufficient folic acid for LBW infants. Folic acid supplementation up to 65 μg/day is, therefore, recommended.

Artificially fed infants

Formulae for LBW infants should provide at least 40 μg of folic acid per dl of reconstituted feed (60 μg/100 kcal). If this is not possible, owing to technical difficulties, then supplementation is recommended up to 65 μg/day. An upper limit cannot be set.

VITAMIN B$_{12}$

Nutritional background

Deficiency of vitamin B$_{12}$ in man causes megaloblastic anaemia, glossitis and neurological symptoms (1,184). Vitamin B$_{12}$ deficiency has not been described in breast-fed infants, with the rare exception of a few infants of women with severe vitamin B$_{12}$ deficiency or on a strictly vegetarian diet (184,211,212).

Toxicity from vitamin B$_{12}$ has not been reported (184).

Available foods

Human milk contains about 0.1 μg/dl of vitamin B$_{12}$ (24,213). Cow's milk has a much higher content (0.3 μg/dl) (7,24). Vitamin B$_{12}$ content of proprietary formulae is extremely variable (0.1–2 μg/dl) but always higher than that of human milk.

Requirements and advisable intakes

Vitamin B$_{12}$ requirements are probably very small, in the order of 0.1–0.5 μg/day (1,184). Normal breast-fed infants receive about 0.3 μg of vitamin B$_{12}$ per day with human milk and this amount has been recommended as an adequate allowance (1,184).

Proprietary formulae for LBW infants should contain at least as much vitamin B$_{12}$ as human milk (0.1 μg/dl).

An upper limit cannot be set.

Summary of guidelines

Infants fed breast milk

There is no evidence that LBW infants fed human milk need to be supplemented with vitamin B$_{12}$.

Artificially fed infants

Proprietary formulae for LBW infants should contain at least 0.1 μg of vitamin B$_{12}$ per dl of reconstituted feed (0.15 μg/100 kcal). An upper limit cannot be set.

VITAMIN C

Vitamin C is easily oxidized in aqueous solution and is inactivated by heat.

Vitamin C activity is usually expressed as μg of L-ascorbic acid. International units are rarely used (1 iu = 50 μg of L-ascorbic acid).

Nutritional background

Ascorbic acid is involved in the hyroxylation of proline and lysine (for collagen synthesis), adrenalin and tryptophane, in the conversion of folic acid into folinic acid, and in the oxidation of tyrosine (214–217). Vitamin C is also important for iron absorption in the gut (216).

Lack of vitamin C causes scurvy in infants; however, the clinical manifestations of vitamin C deficiency usually appear beyond the neonatal period, since tissue reserves at birth are generally good and can counterbalance inadequate dietary intakes (218).

Subclinical vitamin C deficiency is likely when the level of vitamin C in leukocytes falls below 100 μg/g (219).

LBW infants fed high protein casein predominant formulae develop transient elevations of plasma and urine tyrosine, phenylalanine and their metabolites (220,221). This is due to the low activity of the enzyme tyrosine amino-transferase (222). A gradual inhibition by its substrate of the second enzyme involved in the oxidation of tyrosine, p-hydroxy-phenyl-pyruvic-acid-oxidase, may also contribute to the hypertyrosinaemia observed in these infants. Since vitamin C functions as a non-specific reducing agent, preventing the inhibition of this latter enzyme by its substrate, supplementation with vitamin C (50–100 mg/day) will often reduce the incidence and the severity of hypertyrosinaemia (223,224). When vitamin C is introduced in excess of requirements it accumulates in the liver and other tissues until saturation occurs and is then excreted in urine or metabolized to CO_2 (216). Toxicity has not been reported in the newborn.

Available foods

Fresh human milk contains about 4 mg vitamin C/dl (7,24). Pasteurization may reduce the vitamin C concentration by 90% (19). Cow's milk has a much lower content (2 mg/dl) (7,24), while proprietary formulae are usually supplemented with vitamin C (5–30 mg/dl).

Requirements and advisable intakes

Some controversy still exists concerning the recommended allowance of vitamin C in preterm infants. Normal breast-fed term infants usually receive about 15–20 mg/day of ascorbic acid, an amount in excess of that shown to prevent scurvy in adults (1). However, sub-optimal maternal vitamin C status, milk storage and heating may lower considerably the vitamin C content of breast milk (19). Proprietary formulae for LBW infants should, therefore, have a vitamin C content equal to or higher than that of human milk (4 mg/dl); however, formula fed LBW infants should probably receive higher amounts than human milk fed infants, possibly in the range of 20–50 mg/day, for the prevention of hypertyrosinaemia and for optimal iron absorption (19).

Summary of guidelines

Infants fed breast milk

LBW infants fed fresh human milk may receive sufficient vitamin C for their requirements. However, since the vitamin C content of human milk, and particularly heat treated human milk is variable, supplementation is indicated with 20 mg/day ascorbic acid.

Artificially fed infants

Proprietary formulae for LBW infants should contain at least 5 mg vitamin C/dl of reconstituted feed (7 mg/100 kcal). When casein predominant formulae are used or when the amount of formula introduced is such that vitamin C ingestion is less than 20 mg/day, supplementation is indicated (20 mg/day). An upper limit cannot be set, but we see no reason to exceed what is present in available formulae (30 mg/dl; 40 mg/100 kcal).

MULTIVITAMIN PREPARATIONS FOR LBW INFANTS

Although still controversial, multiple vitamin preparations are often given to LBW infants in many neonatal units (225). As mentioned before, under normal circumstances vitamin supplementation is only needed for vitamins A,D,K,C and folic acid, while it is debated for vitamins E, B_1, B_2, and B_6 for which the daily intake may become marginal under certain circumstances.

On the other hand, water-soluble vitamins are non-toxic and readily eliminated and thus no harm can derive when they are given in slight excess of minimal requirements. If multivitamin supplementation is used routinely the following recommendations should be followed.

1 The vitamin content of the preparation should be proportioned to the estimated daily need of each individual vitamin. This may be difficult to achieve since the recommended allowances may be expressed on a daily basis (i.e. vitamin A,D,C and folic acid), on a per kg basis (i.e. vitamin E, B_2), or on the basis of another nutrients intake (i.e. vitamin E, B_6). Therefore, a compromise must be achieved avoiding an excess of those vitamins which may produce toxicity (vitamin A,D,E).

2 Hyperosmolar vitamin solutions should be avoided.

3 Vitamin E should be given as a water-soluble, easily absorbable preparation.

4 Folic acid should be given separately or added to the multiple vitamin preparation shortly before administration since it is easily inactivated.

5 The vitamin intake from the multivitamin preparation should be periodically evaluated (and possibly adjusted) in relation to the calculated intake provided by feedings.

6 A reasonably well balanced multivitamin preparation could provide a daily allowance of:

Vitamin A–300 μg; Vitamin D–20 μg; Vitamin E–5 mg; Vitamin K–3 μg;
Vitamin B_1–50 μg; Vitamin B_2–200 μg; Vitamin B_6–100 μg;
Vitamin C–20 mg;

and folic acid (added or separate)– 60 μg. Niacin, biotin and pantothenic acid need not be included.

Even if a baby up to 2 kg body weight was to receive 165 kcal/kg per day of a formula containing the recommended upper limits of vitamins, the addition of this daily supplement would not be toxic. When the baby has reached 2 kg the total vitamin intake should be reconsidered.

REFERENCES

1. Fomon S.J. (1974). *Infant Nutrition*, 2nd edn. W.B. Saunders, Philadelphia.

2. American Academy of Pediatrics: Committee on Nutrition (1976). Commentary on breast-feeding and infant formulas, including proposed standards for formulas. *Pediatrics* 57, 278–85.
3. American Academy of Pediatrics: Committee on Nutrition (1977). Nutritional needs of low-birth-weight infants. *Pediatrics* **60**, 519–30.
4. ESPGAN: Committee on Nutrition (1977). Guidelines on infant nutrition-1. Recommendation for the composition of an adapted formula. *Acta Paediatr. Scand.* (Suppl.) **262**.
5. Committee on Dietary Allowances, Food and Nutrition Boad, National Research Council (1980). *Recommended Dietary Allowances*, Ninth revised edition. National Academy of Sciences, Washington DC.
6. American Academy of Pediatrics: Committee on Nutrition (1980). Vitamin and mineral supplement needs in normal children in the United States. *Pediatrics* **66**, 1015–21.
7. Department of Health and Social Security, Report on Health and Social Subjects No 18 (1982). *Artificial Feeds for the Young Infant*. HMSO, London.
8. Canadian Paediatric Society, Nutrition Committee. (1981). Feeding the low-birth-weight infant. *CMA J.* **124**, 1301–1311.
9. Orzalesi M. (1982). Do breast and bottle fed babies require vitamin supplements? *Acta Paediatr. Scand.* (Suppl.) **293**, 77–82.
10. Tsang R.C. (1985). Determining the vitamin and mineral requirements in preterm infants: An introduction. In: *Vitamin and Mineral Requirements in Preterm Infants* (ed. R.C. Tsang) pp 1–8. Marcel Dekker, New York.
11. Beaton G.H. (1985). Nutritional needs during the first year of life. Some concepts and perspectives. *Pediatr. Clin. North Am.* **32**, 275–88.
12. American Academy of Pediatrics. Committee on Nutrition (1985). Nutritional needs of low birth weight infants. *Pediatrics* 75, 976–86.
13. Churella H.R., Bachhubez W.K. & MacLean W.C. (1985). Survey: Methods of feeding low birth weight infants. *Pediatrics* 76, 243–9.
14. Marlone J.L. (1975). Vitamin passage across the placenta. *Clin. Perinatol.* 2, 295–307.
15. Farrell P.M., Zachman R.D. & Gutcher G.R. (1985). Fat-soluble vitamins A,E, and K in the premature infant. In: *Vitamin and Mineral Requirements in Preterm Infants* (ed. R.C. Tsang) pp 63–98. Marcel Dekker, New York.
16. Greer F. & Tsang R.C. (1985). Calcium, phosphorus, magnesium and vitamin D requirements for the preterm infants. In: *Vitamin and Mineral Requirements in Preterm Infants* (ed. R.C. Tsang) pp 99–136. Marcel Dekker, New York.
17. Mino M. & Nishino H. (1973). Fetal and maternal relationship in serum vitamin E level. *J. Nutr. Sci. Vitaminol.* **19**, 475–82.
18. Baker H., Frank O., Thomson A.D., Langer A., Munves E.D., De Angelis B. & Kaminetzky H.A. (1975) Vitamin profile of 174 mothers and newborns at parturition. *Am. J. Clin. Nutr.* **28**, 59–65.
19. Schanler R.J. & Nichols B.L. (1985). The water-soluble vitamins C, B_1, B_2, B_6, niacin. In: *Vitamin and Mineral Requirements in Preterm Infants.* (ed. R.C. Tsang) pp 39–62. Marcel Dekker, New York.
20. Raiha N. (1958). On the placental transfer of vitamin C. *Acta Physiol. Scand.* (Suppl) 155.
21. Macy I.G. (1949). Composition of human colostrum and milk. *Am. J. Dis. Child.* **78**, 589.
22. Kon S.K. & Mawson F.H. (1950). *Human milk. Special Report Series of the Medical Research Council* **269**. HMSO, London.
23. Macy I.G. & Kelly H.J. (1961). Human and Cow's milk in infant nutrition. In: *Milk, the Mammary Gland and its Secretions.* (eds. S.K. Kon & A.T. Cokie) p. 265. Academic Press, New York.
24. Department of Health and Social Security, Report on Health and Social Subjects No 12

25. Packard V.S. (1982). *Human milk and Infant Formula*, pp 29–49. Academic Press, New York.

26. Lammi-Keefe C.J. & Jensen R.G. (1984). Fat soluble vitamins in human milk. *Nutr. Rev.* **42**, 365–70.

27. Thompson S.Y., Henry K.M. & Kon S.K. (1964). Factors affecting the concentration of vitamins in milk. I: Effect of breed, season and geographical location on fat soluble vitamins. *J. Dairy Res.* **31**, 1.

28. Ford J.E., Hurrel R.F. & Finot P.A. (1983). Storage of milk powders under adverse conditions. 2: Influence on the content of water-soluble vitamins. *Br. J. Nutr.* **49**, 355–64.

29. Goodman D.S. (1969). Retinol transport in human plasma. *Am. J. Clin. Nutr.* **22**, 911–12.

30. Ong D.E. (1985). Vitamin A-binding proteins. *Nutr. Rev.* **43**, 225–32.

31. Takahaski Y.I., Smith J.E. & Goodman D.S. (1977). Vitamin A and retinol-binding protein metabolism during fetal development in the rat. *Am. J. Physiol.* **233**, 263–4.

32. Vahlquist A., Rask L., Peterson R.A. & Berg T. (1975). The concentration of retinol-binding protein, prealbumin and transferrin in the sera of newly delivered mothers and children of various ages. *Scand. J. Clin. Lab. Invest.* **35**, 569–74.

33. Baker H., Thind I.S., Frank O. *et al.* (1977). Vitamin levels in low birth weight newborn infants and their mothers. *Am. J. Obstet. Gynecol.* **123**, 521–4.

34. Brandt R.B., Mueller D.G., Schroeder J.R. *et al.* (1978). Serum vitamin A in premature and term neonates. *J. Pediatr.* **92**, 101–4.

35. Montreewasuwat N. & Olsen J.A. (1979). Serum and liver concentrations of vitamin A in Thai fetuses as a function of gestational age. *Am. J. Clin. Nutr.* **32**, 601–4.

36. Shenai J.P., Chytil F., Jhaveri A. & Stahlman M.T. (1981). Plasma vitamin A and retinol-binding protein in premature and term neonates. *J. Pediatr.* **99**, 302–5.

37. Woodruff C., Latham C. & James E. (1982). Serum vitamin A in low birth weight infants. *J. Am. Coll. Nutr.* **1**, 125.

38. Moskowitz S.R., Pereira G.R., Heaf L. *et al.* (1982). Retinol-binding protein levels in premature infants: Effect of nutrient intake. *Pediatr. Res.* **16**, 301A.

39. Bhatia J. & Ziegler E.E. (1983). Retinol-binding protein and prealbumin in cord blood of term and preterm infants. *Early Hum. Dev.* **8**, 123–33.

40. Persson B., Tunnel R. & Ekegren K. (1965). Chronic vitamin A intoxication during the first half year of life: description of 5 cases. *Acta Paediatr. Scand.* **54**, 49–52.

41. Shenai J.P., Chytil F. & Stahlman H.P. (1985). Liver vitamin A reserves in very low birth weight neonates. *Pediatr. Res.* **19**, 892–3.

42. Hustead V.A., Gutcher G.R., Anderson S.A. & Zachman R.D. (1984). Relationship of vitamin A (retinol) status to lung disease in the preterm infant. *J. Pediatr.* **105**, 610–15.

43. Shenai J.P., Chytil F. & Stahlman M.T. (1985). Vitamin A status of neonates with bronchopulmonary dysplasia. *Pediatr. Res.* **19**, 185–9.

44. Macy I.G. & Kelly H.J. (1961) Human and cows milk in infant nutrition. In: *Milk the Mammary Gland and its Secretions* (eds S.K. Kon & A.T. Cokie) p. 265. Academic Press, New York.

45. Rodriguez M.S. & Irwin M.I. (1972). A conspectus of research on vitamin A requirements in man. *J. Nutr.* **102**, 909.

46. Bouillon R. & Van Baelen H. (1980). Vitamin D transport. *Acta Paediatr. Belg.* **33**, 3–7.

47. DeLuca H.F. (1979). Vitamin metabolism and function. In: *Monographs on Endocrinology*, Vol. 13 (eds F. Gross, M.M. Grumbach, A. Labhart *et al.*) Springer Verlag, New York.

48. DeLuca H.F. (1980). Some new concepts emanating from a study of the metabolism and function of vitamin D. *Nutr. Rev.* **38**, 169–82.

49. Scully R.E., ed. (1986). Normal references values. *N. Engl. J. Med.* **1**, 39–49.

50. Glorieux F.H., Salle B., Delvin E.E. & David L. (1981). Vitamin D metabolism in preterm infants: its relation to early neonatal hypocalcemia. *In: Intensive Care in the Newborn III.* (eds L. Stern & B. Salle) pp. 127–34. Masson, New York.

51. Atkinson S.A. (1983). Calcium and Phosphorus requirements of low birth weight infants: a nutritional and endocrinological perspective. *Nutr. Rev.* **41**, 69–78.

52. Delvin E., Gloieux F., Salle B., David L. & Varenne J. (1982). Control of vitamin D metabolism in preterm infants: fetomaternal relationships. *Arch Dis. Child.* **57**, 754–7.

53. Hillman L. & Haddad J. (1974). Human perinatal vitamin D metabolism I: 25-Hydroxy-vitamin D in maternal and cord blood. *J. Pediatr.* **84**, 742–9.

54. Weisman Y., Occhipinti M., Knox G., Reiter E. & Root A. (1978). Concentrations of 24, 25-dihyroxyvitamin D and 25-hydroxyvitamin D in paired maternal and cord sera. *Am. J. Obstet. Gynecol.* **130**, 704–7.

55. Wieland P., Fisher J., Trechsel U., Roth H., Vetter K., Schneider H. & Huch A. (1980). Perinatal parthyroid hormone, vitamin D metabolites and calcitonin in man. *Am. J. Physiol.* **239**, 385–90.

56. Gertner J., Glassman M., Coustan D., & Goodman D. (1980). Fetomaternal vitamin D relationships at term. *J. Pediatr.* **97**, 637–40.

57. Verity C., Burman D., Beadle P., Holton J. & Morris A. (1981). Seasonal changes in perinatal vitamin D metabolism: maternal and cord blood biochemistry in normal pregnancies. *Arch Dis. Child.* **56**, 943–8.

58. Bouillon R., Van Assche F., Van Baelen H., Heyns W., & De Moor P. (1981). Influence of the vitamin D-binding protein on the serum concentration of 1,25-dihydroxyvitamin D_3. Significance of the free 1,25-dihydroxyvitamin D concentration. *J. Clin. Invest.* **67**, 589–96.

59. Tsang R.C., Greer F. & Steichen J.J. (1981). Perinatal metabolism of vitamin D: Transition from fetal to neonatal life. *Clin. Perinatol.* **8**, 287–306.

60. Seino Y., Ishida M., Yamaoka K., Ishii T., Hiejima T., Ikehara C., Tanaka Y., Matsuda S., Shimotsuji T., Yabuuchi H., Morimoto S. & Onishi T. (1982). Serum calcium regulating hormones in the perinatal period. *Calcif. Tissue Int.* **54**, 131–5.

61. Tsang R.C. (1983). The quandary of vitamin D in the newborn infant. *Lancet* i, 1370–2.

62. Tsang R.C., Steichen J.J. & Brown D.R. (1979). Perinatal calcium homeostasis: neonatal hypocalcaemia and bone demineralization. *Clin. Perinat.* **4**, 385–409.

63. Wolf H., Graff V. & Offerman G. (1979). The vitamin D requirements for premature infants. In: *Vitamin D Bone and its Clinical Application* (eds A. Norman, K. Schaefer, D. Herrath & H. Grigoleit, pp. 349–52. Walter de Gruyter, Berlin.

64. Glorieux F., Salle B., Delvin E. & David L. (1981). Vitamin D metabolism in preterm infants: serum calcitriol values during the first five days of life. *J. Pediatr.* **99**, 640–3.

65. Robinson M., Merrett A., Tetlow V. & Compston J. (1981). Plasma 25-hydroxyvitamin D concentrations in preterm infants receiving oral vitamin D supplements. *Arch Dis. Child.* **56**, 144–5.

66. Salle B., David L., Glorieux F., Delvin E., Senterre J. & Renaud H. (1982). The effect of early oral administration of vitamin D and its metabolites in premature neonates on mineral homeostasis. *Pediatr. Res.* **16**, 75–8.

67. Salle B., Glorieux F., Delvin E., David L. & Meunier G. (1983). Vitamin D metabolism in preterm infants. *Acta Paediatr. Scand.* **72**, 203–6.

68. Markstead T., Aksnes L., Finne P. & Aarskog D. (1983). Vitamin D nutritional status of premature infants supplemented with 500 IU vitamin D_2 per day. *Acta Paediatr. Scand.* **73**, 517–20.

69. Markstad T., Aksnes L., Finne P. & Aarskog D. (1984). Plasma concentrations of vitamin D metabolites in premature infants. *Pediatr. Res.* **18**, 269–72.

70. Senterre J., David L. & Salle B. (1981). Effects of 1.25-dihydroxycholecalciferol on calcium, phosphorus and magnesium balance, and on circulating parathyroid hormone and calcitonin in preterm infants. *In: Intensive Care in the Newborn III.* (ed. L. Stern & B. Salle) pp. 115–25. Masson, New York.

71. Senterre J. & Salle B. (1982). Calcium and phosphorus economy of the preterm infant and its interaction with vitamin D and its metabolites. *Acta Paediatr. Scand* (Suppl.) **296**, 85-92.

72. Senterre J., Putet G., Salle B. & Rigo J. (1983). Effects of vitamin D and phosphorus supplementation on calcium retention in preterm infants fed banked human milk. *J. Pediatr.* **103**, 305–7.

73. Seino Y., Ishi T., Shimotsuji T. *et al.* (1981). Plasma active vitamin D concentration in low birth weight infants with rickets and its response to vitamin D treatment. *Arch Dis. Child.* **56**, 628–32.

74. Hillman L.S., Hoff N., Salmons S., *et al.* (1985). Mineral homeostasis in very premature infants: Serial evaluation of serum 25-hydroxyvitamin D, serum minerals and bone mineralization. *J. Pediatr.* **106**, 970–80.

75. Hillman L.S., Hollis B., Salmons S. *et al.* (1985). Absorption, dosage and effect on mineral homeostasis of 25-hydroxycholecalciferol in premature infants: comparison with 400 and 800 i.u. vitamin D_2 supplementation. *J. Pediatr.* **106**, 981–9.

76. Cifuentes R.F., Kooh S.W. & Raddle I.C. (1978). Vitamin D deficiency in very low birth weight infants. *Proc. Can. Fed. Biol. Soc.* **21**, 46A.

77. Finberg L. (1981). Human milk feeding and vitamin D supplementation. *J. Pediatr.* **99**, 228–31.

78. Makin H.L.J., Seamark A. & Trafford J.H. (1983). Vitamin D and its metabolites in human breast milk. *Arch. Dis. Child.* **58**, 750–3.

79. Le Boulch N., Gulat-Marnay C. & Raoul Y. (1974). Dérivéves de la vitamine D_3 des laits de femme et de vache: ester sulfate de cholécalciférol et hydroxy-25-cholécalciférol. *Int. J. Vit. Nutr. Res.* **44**, 167–70.

80. Lakdawala D.R. & Widdowson E.M. (1977). Vitamin D in human milk. *Lancet* **1**, 167–8.

81. Leerbeck E., & Sondergaard H. (1980). The total content of vitamin D in human milk and cow's milk. *Br. J. Nutr.* **44**, 7–12.

82. Brooke O.G. & Lucas A. (1985). Metabolic bone disease in preterm infants. *Arch Dis. Child.* **60**, 682–5.

83. McCay P.B. & King M. (1980). Biochemical function. In: *Vitamin E. A Comprehensive Treatise.* (Ed. L.J. Machlin) pp 289–317. Marcel Dekker, New York.

84. Williams M.L., Shott R.J., O'Neal P.L. & Oski F.A. (1975). Role of dietary iron and fat on vitamin E deficiency anaemia of infancy. *N. Engl. J. Med.* **292**, 887–90.

85. Gross S.J. & Gabriel E. (1985). Vitamin E status in preterm infants fed human milk or infant formula. *J. Pediatr.* **106**, 635–9.

86. Mason H.F. & Filer L.J. Jnr. (1947). Interrelationships of dietary fat and tocopherols. *J. Am. Oil Chem. Soc.* **24**, 240–2.

87. Hashim S.A., Asfour R.I.I. (1968). Tocopherol in infants fed diets rich in polyunsaturated fatty acids. *Am. J. Clin. Nutr.* **21**, 7–14.

88. Witting L.A. (1974). Vitamin E-polyunsaturated lipid relationship in diet and tissues. *Am. J. Clin. Nutr.* **27**, 952–9.

89. Harris P.L. & Embree N.D. (1963). Quantitative consideration of the effect of polyunsaturated fatty acid content of the diet upon the requirements for vitamin E. *Am. J. Clin. Nutr.* **13**, 385–92.

90. Bell E.F. & Filer L.J. (1981). The role of vitamin E in the nutrition of premature infants. *Am. J. Clin. Nutr.* **74**, 414–22.

91. Hassan H., Hashim S.A., Van Itallie T.B. & Sebrell W.H. (1966). Syndrome in premature infants associated with low plasma vitamin E levels and high polyunsaturated fatty acid diet. *Am. J. Clin. Nutr.* **19**, 147–57.

92. Oski F.A. & Barness L.A. (1967). Vitamin E deficiency: a previously unrecognized cause of hemolytic anemia in the premature infant. *J. Pediatr* **70**, 211–20.

93. Ritchie J.H., Fisch M.B., McMasters V. & Grossman M. (1968). Edema and hemolytic

anemia in premature infants: a vitamin E deficiency syndrome. *N. Engl. J. Med.* **279**, 1185–90.

94. Leonard P.J., Doyle E. & Harrington W. (1972). Levels of vitamin E in the plasma of newborn infants and of their mothers. *Am. J. Clin. Nutr.* **25**, 480–5.

95. Moyer W.T. (1950). Vitamin E levels in term and premature newborn infants. *Pediatrics* **6**, 893–6.

96. Wright S.W., Filer L.J. & Mason K.E. (1951). Vitamin E blood levels in premature and full term infants. *Pediatrics* **7**, 386–93.

97. Haga P. & Lunde G. (1978). Selenium and vitamin E in cord blood from preterm and full term infants. *Acta Paediatr. Scand.* **67**, 735–9.

98. Martinez F.E., Goncalves A.L., Jorge S.M. & Desai I.D. (1981). Vitamin E in placental blood and its interrelationship to maternal and newborn levels of vitamin E. *J. Pediatr.* **99**, 298–300.

99. Bieri J.G. & Farrell P.M. (1976). Vitamin E. *Vit. Horm.* **34**, 31–75.

100. Horwitt M.K., Harvey C.C., Dahm C.H. & Searcy M.T. (1972). Relationship between tocopherol and serum lipid levels for determination of nutritional adequacy. *Ann. N.Y. Acad. Sci.* **203**, 223–36.

101. Farrell P.M., Levine S.L., Murphy M.D. & Adam A.J. (1978). Plasma tocopherol levels and tocopherol-lipid relationship in a normal population of children as compared to healthy adults. *Am. J. Clin. Nutr.* **31**, 1720–6.

102. Duc G. & Tuchschmid P. (1986). Use and abuse of vitamin E in the newborn. In: *Proceedings of the International Symposium of Neonatology.* (Eds G. Cucinotta, E. Mazzaglia & M. Orzalesi) pp 255–78. EDAS EDIZ, Messina.

103. Farrel P.M., Mischler E.H. & Guther G.R. (1982). Evaluation of vitamin E deficiency in children with lung disease. *Ann. N.Y. Acad. Sci.* **393**, 96.

104. Sartain P., Kay J.L. & Dorn P.M. (1967). The effect of vitamin E on the early anemia of prematurity. *South Med. J.* **60**, 1371–7.

105. Carina S.D., Cruz P.D., Wimberley K. *et al.* (1983). The effect of vitamin E on erythrocyte hemolysis and lipid peroxidation in newborn premature infants. *Acta Paediatr. Scand.* **72**, 823–6.

106. Horwitt M.K. (1980). Therapeutic uses of vitamin E in medicine. *Nutr. Rev.* **38**, 105–13.

107. Ehrenkranz R.A. (1980). Vitamin E and the neonate. *Am. J. Dis. Child.* **134**, 1157–66.

108. Johnson L., Schaffer D., Quinn D. *et al.* (1982). Vitamin E supplementation and the retinopathy of prematurity. *Ann. N.Y. Acad. Sci.* **393**, 473.

109. Phelps D.L. Vitamin E and Retrolental Fibroplasia in 1982. *Pediatrics* **70**, 420–5.

110. Johnson L., Schaffer D. & Boggs T.R. Jr. (1974). The premature infant, vitamin E deficiency and retrolental fibroplasia. *Am. J. Clin. Nutr.* **27**, 1158–73.

111. Johnson L.H., Schaffer D.B., Rubinstein D., Crawford C.S. & Boggs T.R. (1976). The role of vitamin E in retrolental fibroplasia. *Paediatr. Res.* **10**, 425.

112. Johnson L., Schaffer D., Boggs T., Quinn G. & Mathis M. (1980). Vitamin E rx of retrolental fibroplasia grade III or worse. *Pediatr. Res.* **14**, 601.

113. Kretzer F.L., Hittner H.M., Johnson A.T. *et al.* (1982). Vitamin E and retrolental fibroplasia: ultrastructural support of clinical efficacy. *Ann. N.Y. Acad. Sci.* **393**, 145–58.

114. Hittner H.M., Godio M.D., Rudolph A.J. *et al.* (1981). Retrolental fibroplasia: Efficacy of vitamin E in a double blind clinical study of preterm infants. *N. Engl. J. Med.* **305**, 1365–71.

115. Finer M.N., Schindler R.F., Grant G. *et al.* (1982). Effect of intramuscular vitamin E on the frequency and severity of retrolental fibroplasia: a controlled trial. *Lancet.* **i**, 1087–91.

116. Ehrenkranz R.A., Bonta B.W., Ablow R.C. & Warshaw J.B. (1978). Amelioration of bronchopulmonary dysplasia after vitamin E administration: a preliminary report. *N. Engl. J. Med.* **299**, 564–9.

117. Mc Clung H.J., Backes C., Lavin A. & Kerzner B. (1980). Prospective evaluation of vitamin

118. Ehrenkranz R.A., Ablow R.C. & Warshaw J.B. (1979). Prevention of bronchopulmonary dysplasia with vitamin E administration during the acute stages of respiratory distress syndrome. *J. Pediatr.* **95**, 873–8.

119. Abbasi S, Johnson L. & Boggs T. (1980). Effect of vitamin E by infusion in sick small premature infants at risk for BPD. *Pediatr. Res.* **14**, 638.

120. Saldanha R.L., Cepeda E.E. & Poland R.L. (1980). Effect of prophylactic vitamin E on the development of bronchopulmonary dysplasia in high risk neonates. *Pediatr. Res.* **14**, 650.

121. Finer N.N., Peters K.L., Schindler R.F. & Grant G.D. (1981). Vitamin E, retrolental fibroplasia and bronchopulmonary dysplasia. *Pediatr. Res.* **15**, 660.

122. Watts J.L., Paes B.A., Milner R.A. *et al.* (1981). Randomized controlled trial of vitamin E and bronchopulmonary dysplasia. *Pediatr. Res.* **15**, 686.

123. Chiswick M.L., Wynn J. & Toner N. (1982). Vitamin E and intraventricular haemorrhage in the newborn. *Ann. N.Y. Acad. Sci.* **393**, 109–18.

124. Chiswick M.L., Johnson M., Woodhall C. *et al.* (1983). Protective effect of vitamin E (DL-α-Tocopherol) against intraventricular haemorrhage in premature babies. *Br. Med. J.* **287**, 81–4.

125. Speer M.E., Blifeld C., Rudolph A.J. *et al.* (1984). Intraventricular hemorrhage and vitamin E in the very low birth weight infant: Evidence for efficacy of early intramuscular vitamin E administration. *Pediatrics* **74**, 1107–12.

126. Phelps D.L. (1984). Vitamin E and CNS hemorrhage. *Pediatrics* **74**, 1113–14.

127. Jansen R.D. (1985). Questions on the vitamin E study (letter). *Pediatrics* **76**, 326–7.

128. Melhorn D.K., Gross S. & Childers G. (1979). Vitamin E dependent anemia in the premature infant. I. Effects of large doses of medicinal iron. *J. Pediatr.* **79**, 569–80.

129. Fermanian J., Salomon D., Olive G., Zambroski S., Rossier A. & Caldera R. (1976). Vitamin E versus placebo: a double blind comparative trial in the low birth weight infant in the seventh week of life. *Nouv. Rev. Fr. Hematol.* **16**, 246–53.

130. Jansson L., Holmberf L., Milsson B. & Johansson B. (1978). Vitamin E requirements of preterm infants. *Acta Paediatr. Scand.* **67**, 459–63.

131. Gross S. & Melhorn D.K. (1974). Vitamin E dependent anaemia in the premature infant. III: Comparative hemoglobin, Vitamin E, and erythrocyte phospholipid responses following absorption of either water-soluble or fat-soluble d-α-tocopherol. *J. Pediatr.* **85**, 753–60.

132. Goldbloom R.B. (1963). Studies of tocopherol requirements in health and disease. *Pediatrics* **32**, 36–45.

133. Panos T.C., Stinnett B., Zapata G., Emminians J., Margasigan B.V. & Beard A.G. (1968). Vitamin E and linoleic acid in the feeding of premature infants. *Am. I. Clin. Nutr.* **21**, 15–39.

134. Gross S.J., Landaw S.A. & Oski F.A. (1977). Vitamin E and neonatal hemolysis *Pediatrics* **59**, 995–7.

135. Blanchette V., Bell E., Nahmias C., Garnett S., Milner R. & Zipursky A. (1980). A randomized control trial of vitamin E therapy in the prevention of anemia in low birth weight infants. *Pediatr. Res.* **14**, 591.

136. Chadd M.A. & Fraser A.J. (1970). A controlled trial of vitamin E therapy in infancy. *Int. J. Vit. Res.* **40**, 610–16.

137. Farrell P.M. & Bieri J.C. (1975). Megavitamin E supplementation in man. *Am. J. Clin. Nutr.* **28**, 1281–6.

138. Zipursky A., Milner R.A., Blanchette V.S. & Johnston M.A. (1980). The effects of vitamin E therapy on blood coagulation tests in newborn infants. *Pediatrics* **66**, 547–50.

139. Johnson L., Bower F.W., Abbasi S. *et al.* (1985). Relationship of prolonged pharmacologic serum levels of vitamin E to incidence of sepsis and necrotizing entercolitis in infants with birth weight 1500 grams or less. *Pediatrics* **75**, 618–38.

140. Phelps D.L. (1984). E-Ferol: what happened and what now? *Pediatrics* **74**, 1114–16.

141. Bucher J.R. & Roberts R.J. (1981). Alpha tocopherol (Vitamin E) content of lung, liver, and

blood in the newborn rat and human infant: Influence of hyperoxia. *J. Pediatr.* **98**, 806–11.

142. Hittner H.M. (1984). Reply to a letter to the Editor. *Pediatrics* **74**, 565-9.

143. Finer N.N., Peters K.L., Hayek Z. *et al.* (1984). Vitamin E and necrotizing entercolitis. *Pediatrics* **73**, 387.

144. Bodenstein C.J. (1984). Intravenous vitamin E and deaths in the intensive care unit; letter. *Pediatrics* **73**, 733.

145. Lorch V., Murphy O., Hoersten L.R. *et al.* (1985). Unusual syndrome among premature infants: Association with a new intravenous vitamin E product. *Pediatrics* **75**, 598–602.

146. Melhorn P.K., Gross S. & Childers G. (1971). Vitamin E-dependent anemia in the premature infant. II. relationships between gestational age and absorption of vitamin E. *J. Pediatr.* **79**, 581–8.

147. Filer L.J., Wright S.W., Manning M.P. & Mason K.E. (1951). Absorption of ∝tocopheryl esters by premature and full term infants and children in health and disease. *Pediatrics* **8**, 328–39.

148. Bell E.F., Brown E.J., Milner R., Sinclair J.C. & Zipursky A. (1979). Vitamin E absorption in small premature infants. *Pediatrics* **63**, 830–2.

149. Jansson L., Lindroth M. & Työppönen J. (1984). Intestinal absorption of vitamin E in low birth weight infants. *Acta Paediatr. Scand.* **73**, 329–32.

150. Hittner H.M., Spcer M.E., Rudolph A.J. *et al.* (1984). Retrolental fibroplasia and vitamin E in the pre-term infant — Comparison of oral versus intramuscular:oral administration. *Pediatrics* **73**, 238–49.

151. American Academy of Pediatrics — Committee on the Fetus and Newborn (1985). Vitamin E and the prevention of retinopathy of prematurity. *Pediatrics* **76**, 315–16.

152. Dam H., Dyggve H., Larsen H. & Plum P. (1952). The relation of vitamin K deficiency to haemorrhagic disease of the newborn. *Adv. Pediatr.* **5**, 129–38.

153. Goldman H.J. & Desposito F. (1966). Hypoprothrombinemic bleeding in young infants associated with diarrhoea, antibiotics, and milk substitutes. *Am. J. Dis. Child.* **111**, 430–6.

154. American Academy of Pediatrics Committee on Nutrition (1961). Vitamin K compounds and the water-soluble analogues: use in therapy and prophylaxis in pediatrics. *Pediatrics* **28**, 500.

155. American Academy of Pediatrics-Committee on Nutrition (1971). Vitamin K supplementation for infants receiving milk substitute infant formulas and for those with fat malabsorption. *Pediatrics* **48**, 483.

156. Bjornsson T.D., Meffin P.J., Smezey S.E. & Blascke T.F. (1980). Disposition and turnover of vitamin K_1 in man. In: *Vitamin K Metabolism and Vitamin K-Dependent Proteins* (ed J.W. Suttie). pp 328–32. University Park Press, Baltimore.

157. Lefevere M.F., DeLeeheer A.P. & Claeys A.E. (1979). High-performance liquid chromatography assay of vitamin K in human serum. *J. Chromatogr.* **186**, 749–62.

158. Shearer M.J., Barkhan P., Rahim S. & Stimmler. L. (1982). Plasma vitamin K in mothers and their newborn babies. *Lancet* **i**, 460–3.

159. Corrigan J.J. (1981). The vitamin K-dependent proteins. *Adv. Pediatr.* **28**, 57–74.

160. Suzuki S. (1979). Studies on coagulation in newborn infants: Liver maturation and vitamin K precoagulant-inhibitor relations. *J. Perinat. Med.* **7**, 229–32.

161. Corrigan J.J. Jr. & Krye J.J. (1980). Factor II (prothrombin) levels in cord blood: Correlation of coagulant activity with immunoreactive protein. *J. Pediatr.* **97**, 979–83.

162. Lane P.A., Hathaway W.E., Githens J.H. *et al.* (1983). Fatal intracranial hemorrhage in a normal infant secondary to vitamin K deficiency. *Pediatrics* **72**, 562–4.

163. Von Kries R., Shearer M.J. & McCarthy P.T. (1985). Vitamin K deficiency in breast fed infants (letter). *J. Pediatr.* **107**, 650–1.

164. Von Kries R., Masse B., Becker A. & Gobel U. (1985). Late vitamin K deficiency in healthy infants? (letter). *Lancet* **ii**, 1421–2.

165. Anonymous (editorial) (1985). Late onset of haemorrhagic disease of the newborn. *Nutr. Rev.* **43**, 303–5.

166. Lane P.A. & Hathaway W.E. (1985). Vitamin K in infancy. *J. Pediatr* **106**, 351–9.

167. Owens C.A. Jr. (1971). Pharmacology and toxicology of the vitamin K group. *The Vitamins*, Vol. 3 (eds W.H. Sebrell and R.S. Harris) pp 492–509). Academic, New York.

168. Haroon Y., Shearer M.J., Rahim S. *et al.* (1980). The content of Phylloquinone (vit. K_1) in human milk, cow's and infant formula foods determined by high-performance liquid chromatography. *J. Nutr.* **112**, 1105.

169. Schneider D.L., Fluckinger H.B. & Manes J.D. (1974). Vitamin K_2 content of infant formula products. *Pediatrics* **53**, 273.

170. McNish A.W., Upton C., Samuels M. *et al.* (1985). Plasma concentrations after oral or intramuscular vitamin K_1 in neonates. *Arch. Dis. Child.* **60**, 814–18.

171. Droese W. & Stolley H. (1982). Thiaminbilanz des Säuglings in 1 Lebensviertieljahr-ein Hinweis für den Bedarf. In: *Sanglingsernahron Heute*. (ed. R. Gruttner) pp 66–73. Springer-Verlag, Berlin.

172. Macy I.G., Kelly H.J. & Sloan R.E. (1953). *The Composition of Milks*. National Research Council Publications No 254. Nat. Acad. Sci. Washington.

173. Holt I.E. Jr. Nemir R.L., Synderman W.E. *et al.* (1949). The thiamine requirement of the normal infant. *J. Nutr.* **37**, 53–66.

174. Leboulanger J. (1981). *Le Vitamine*. A. Mondadori, Milan.

175. Lucas A. & Bates C (1984). Transient riboflavin depletion in preterm infants. *Arch. Dis. Child.* **59**, 837–41.

176. Hovi L., Hekali R. & Siimes M.A. (1979). Evidence of riboflavin depletion in breast fed newborns and its further acceleration during treatment of hyperbilirubinemia by phototherapy. *Acta Paediatr. Scand.* **68**, 567–70.

177. Coursin D.B. (1954). Convulsive seizures in infants with pyridoxine-deficient diet. *J. Am. Med. Ass.* **154**, 406–10.

178. Reiken L. (1982). *Ermittlung des vitamin B₆-Bedarfs bei Neugeborenen un jungen Sauglingsnahrung heute*. pp 74–81. Springer-Verlag, Berlin.

179. Gross S.J. (1985). Choline, Pantothenic Acid, and Biotin. In: *Vitamin and Mineral Requirements in Preterm Infants* (ed. R.C. Tsang) p 185–201. Marcel Dekker, New York.

180. Gompertz D., Graffain D.M., Watts J.L. & Hull D. (1971). Biotine responsible ∝-methylcrotonylglycinuria. *Lancet* **ii**, 22–4.

181. Burri B.J., Sweetman L. & Nyham W.L. (1981). Mutant holocarboxylase synthetase. Evidence for the enzyme defect in early infantile biotin-responsive multiple carboxylase deficiency. *J. Clin. Invest.* **68**, 1491–4.

182. Mock D.M., De Losimer A.A., Liebman W.M., Sweetman L. & Baker H. (1981). Biotin deficiency: an unusual complication of parental alimentation. *N. Engl. J. Med.* **304**–320.

183. Kien C.L., Kohler E., Goodman S.I., Berlow S., Hong R., Horowitz S.P. & Baker H. Biotin responsive in vivo carboxylase deficiency in two siblings with secretory diarrhea receiving total parenteral nutrition. *J. Pediatr.* **99**, 546–9.

184. Ek J. (1985). Folic acid and vitamin B_{12} requirements in premature infants. In: *Vitamin and Mineral Requirements in Preterm Infants*. (ed. R.C. Tsang). Marcel Dekker, New York. pp. 23–38.

185. Matoth Y., Zehavi I., Topper E. & Klein T. (1979). Folate nutrition and growth in infancy *Arch. Dis. Child.* **54**, 699.

186. Gandy G & Jacobson W. (1977). Influence of folic acid on birth weight and growth of the erythroblastotic infant. II Growth during the first year. *Arch. Dis. Child.* **52**, 7.

187. Matoth Y., Zamir R., Bar-Shani S. & Grossowicz N. (1964). Studies on folic acid in infancy. II Folic and folinic acid blood levels in infants with diarrhea, malnutrition and infection.

Pediatrics **33**, 694.

188. Gordon S.J. (1974) Anticonvulsive drugs increase the need for folic acid. Quoted by Fomon.

189. Dallman P.R. (1974). Iron, vitamin E and folate in the preterm infant. *J. Pediatr.* **85**, 742–5.

190. Shojania A.M. & Hornaday G. (1970). Folate metabolism in newborns and during early infancy. II. Clearance of folic acid in plasma and excretion of folic acid in urine by newborns. *Pediatr. Res.* **4**, 422.

191. Ek J. (1980). Plasma and red cell folate values in newborn infants and their mothers in relation to gestational age. *J. Pediatr.* **97**, 288.

192. Gray O.P. & Butler E.B. (1965). Megaloblastic anaemia in premature infants. *Arch. Dis. Child.* **40**, 53—7.

193. Roberts P.M., Arrowsmith D.E., Rau S.M. & Monk-Jones M.E. (1969). Folate state of premature infants. *Arch. Dis. Child.* **44**, 637.

194. Strelling M.K., Blackledge D.G. & Goodall H.B. (1979). Diagnosis and management of folate deficiency in low-birth-weight infants. *Arch. Dis. Child.* **54**, 271.

195. Herbert V. (1962). Experimental nutritional folate deficiency in man. *Trans. Ass. Am. Phys.* **75**, 307.

196. Hoffbran A.V. (1970). Folate deficiency in premature infants. *Arch. Dis. Child.* **45**, 441.

197. Kendall A.C., Jones E.E., Wilson C.I.D. *et al.* (1974). Folic acid in low-birth-weight infants. *Arch. Dis. Child.* **49**, 736.

198. Vanner T.M. & Tyas J.F. (1967). Folic acid status in premature infants. *Arch. Dis. Child.* **42**, 57.

199. Stevens D., Burman D., Strelling M.K. & Morris A. (1979). Folic acid supplementation in low-birth weight infants. *Pediatrics* **64**, 333.

200. Roberts P.M.M., Arrowsmith D.E., Lloyd A.V.C. & Monk-Jones M.E. (1972). Effect of folic acid treatment on premature infants. *Arch. Dis. Child.* **47**, 631–4.

201. Burland W.L., Simpson K. & Lord J. (1971). Response of low birth weight infants to treatment with folic acid. *Arch. Dis. Child.* **46**, 189.

202. Kamen B.A. & Caston J.D. (1975). Purification of folate binding factor in normal umbilical cord serum. *Proc. Natl. Acad. Sci.* **73**, 4261.

203. Fernades-Costa F. & Metz J. (1981). The specific folate-binding capacity of serum. Evidence that levels are not directly related to folate nutrition but influenced by hormonal status. *J. Lab. Clin. Med.* **98**, 119.

204. Ford J.E. & Scott K.J. (1968). The folic acid activity of some milk foods for babies. *J. Dairy Res.* **35**, 85.

205. Tamura T., Yoshimura Y. & Arakawa T. (1980). Human milk folate and folate status in lactating mothers and their infants. *Am. J. Clin. Nutr.* **33**, 193.

206. Cooperman J.M., Dueck H.S., Newman L.J. *et al.* (1982). The folate in human milk. *Am. J. Clin. Nutr.* **36**, 576.

207. Karlin R. (1966). Sur le variations de taux d'acide folique total dans le lait de femme au cours de la lactation. Comparison aven le lait bovin. *Compt. Rend. Soc. Biol.* (Paris) **160**, 2123.

208. Causeret J. (1979). Vitamin value of an animal milk compared to that of human milk. *Ann. Nutr. Aliment.* **2**, A 313.

209. Ek J. & Magnus E. (1982). Plasma and red cell folate values and folate requirements in formula fed term infants. *J. Pediatr.* **100**, 738.

210. Ek J. & Magnus E. (1979). Plasma and red blood cell folate in breast fed infants. *Acta Paediatr. Scand.* **68**, 239.

211. Lampkin B.C., Shore N.A. & Chadwick D. (1966). Megaloblastic anaemia of infancy secondary to maternal pernicious anaemia. *N. Engl. J. Med.* **274**, 1168–71.

212. Higginbottom M.C., Sweetman L. & Nyham W.L. (1978). Syndrome of methylmalonic aciduria, homocystinuria, megaloblastic anaemia and neurologic abnormalities in vitamin B_{12}—deficient breast fed infant of a strict vegetarian. *N. Engl. J. Med.* **299**, 317–23.

213. Sandberg D.P., Begley J.A. & Hall C.A. (1981). The content, binding and forms vitamin B$_{12}$ in milk. *Am. J. Child. Nutr.* **34**, 1717.
214. Prockop D.J. & Guzman N.A. (1977). Collagen diseases and the biosynthesis of collagen. *Hosp. Pract.* **12**, 61–8.
215. Mussie E.A. (1967). Collagen formation. *Science* **157**, 927–9.
216. Moran J.R. & Green H.L. (1979). The vitamins and vitamin C in human nutrition. *Am. J. Dis. Child.* **133**, 308–14.
217. Stokes P.L., Melikian V. & Leeming R.L. (1975). Folate metabolism in scurvy. *Am. J. Clin. Nutr.* **28**, 126–9.
218. Ingalls T.H. (1938). Ascorbic acid requirements in early infancy. *N. Engl. J. Med.* **218**, 872–5.
219. Sauberlich H.E. (1977). Vitamin C status: Methods and findings. *Ann. N.Y. Acad. Sci.* **258**, 438–50.
220. La Du B.N. & Gjessing L.R. (1978). Tyrosinosis and tyrosinemia. In: *Metabolic Basis of Inherited Disease.* (ed. J.B. Salsbury, J.B. Wyngaarden & D.S. Fredrickson) p. 256. McGraw Hill, New York.
221. Rassin D.K., Gaull G.E., Raiha N.C.R. & Heinonen K. (1977). Milk protein quantity and quality in low-birth-weight-infants. IV. Effect on tyrosine and phenylalanine in plasma and urine. *J. Pediatr.* **90**, 356–60.
222. Anderson S,M., Raiha N.C.R. & Ohiselo J.J. (1980). Tyrosine aminotransferase activity in human fetal liver. *J. Develop. Physiol.* **2**, 17–27.
223. Levine S.Z., Gordon H.H. & Marples E. (1941). Defect in the metabolism of tyrosine and phenylalanine in premature infants. II. Spontaneous occurrence and eradication by vitamin C. *J. Clin. Invest.* **20**, 209.
224. Synderman S.E. (1971). The protein and aminoacid requirements of the premature infant. In: (eds J.P.H. Jonxis, H.R.A. Visser, J.A. Troelstra) *Metabolic Processes in the Fetus and Newborn Infant.* H.E. Stenfert Kroese N.V., Leiden.
225. Pereira G.R. & Barbosa N.M.M. (1986). Controversies in neonatal nutrition. *Pediatr. Clin. N. Am.* **33** (1), 65–89.

8
Sodium, Potassium and Chloride

SODIUM

Nutritional background

Sodium is present in the body in both ionized and bound forms. In the newborn, estimates of exchangeable sodium are about 96% of total body sodium determined by carcass analysis, so firmly bound sodium is a relatively small proportion of total body sodium in newborn infants(1). The exchangeable sodium is the main cation of the extracellular fluid and contributes to many of its physical properties. The amount and concentration of sodium in the extracellular fluid (ECF) determines the volume and contributes to its osmotic activity, while the sodium:potassium gradient across cell membranes generated by sodium:potassium ATPase provides the energy gradient that drives most membrane transport processes, and the propagation of the nerve and muscle action potential. It acts as a counter substituting ion in acid base regulation and contributes to the stability of proteins and of membranes.

Sodium in the fetal body

The sodium concentration of the fetal body falls from about 94 mmol/kg at 25 weeks gestation (500 g body weight) to about 74 mmol/kg at term (3.5 kg body weight) (1,2). The daily rate of accumulation of sodium by the fetus differs slightly depending on how it is calculated (2,3) but is probably in the range 0.85–1.1 mmol/kg per day. Such estimates give some idea of a sodium retention that would be satisfactory in a growing preterm infant, but because of the problems of renal sodium handling experienced by these babies (vide infra) the intrauterine accumulation rate cannot be used alone to estimate the optimal dietary sodium intake.

Sodium deficiency

Sodium depletion may be associated with a proportionate loss of water in which case there will be isotonic dehydration and the signs will predominantly be those of contraction of ECF volume leading to renal failure. Sodium depletion by itself will lead to hypotonicity of the ECF, hyponatraemia, and a shift of water into the cells. If it is severe, the signs of water intoxication will develop.

Though sodium deficiency may have secondary effects on growth (e.g. through blood volume reduction impairing the microcirculation) there is no firm evidence at present that linear or soft tissue growth are materially impaired if the plasma sodium is maintained above 130 mmol/l.

Changes in sodium balance following birth and the causes of hyponatraemia

The first week
Preterm infants lose weight during the first week following birth (4) and this is associated with a loss of sodium, reported to be between 6 and 16 mmol sodium/kg body weight (5). This negative balance occurs in spite of positive nitrogen and potassium balance (5), and is probably independent of sodium intake in the range 1–6 mmol/kg per day (4,5,6). The proportion of body sodium lost is greatest in the most immature infants, and from changes in sodium balance and in body weight it can be estimated that 70–80% of the weight loss seen in infants of about 1.0 kg birth weight is due to isotonic loss of ECF (6). Since the ECF of the fetus is thought to fall from about 60% of body weight at 26 weeks of gestation to about 40% at term (7), the estimated loss of ECF by preterm infants after birth would result in a ratio of ECF to ICF more resembling though not the same as that of a full term infant. Though a small increase in sodium intake may be needed towards the end of the first week of life in some infants with excess weight loss and hyponatraemia, it must be recognized that the commonest cause of hyponatraemia during the first four to five days of life is probably water retention secondary to inappropriate secretion of antidiuretic hormone (8, 9).

The second and subsequent weeks
Most reports indicate that sodium balance is positive by the 7th–11th day of life. For example, six infants of <1.5 kg birth weight studied sequentially between the 10th and 70th day of life on an intake of 2.3 mmolNa$^+$/kg per day, absorbed on average 1.9 mmolNa$^+$/kg per day and retained 1.1 mmolNa$^+$/kg per day, a value close to the estimated intrauterine accumulation rate (10). Day *et al* (1976) (11) also found preterm infants receiving 1.6–1.7 mmol/kg per day to be in positive balance between 14 and 49 days of life at a time when there was a high incidence of hyponatraemia (<130 mmolNa$^+$/l). They were able to correct this 'late hyponatraemia' by increasing sodium intake to 3.0 mmol/kg per day (12). According to Gross (1983) (13) late hyponatraemia (<133

mmolNa$^+$/l after the first week of life) developed in 50% of infants fed pooled breast milk providing 1.3 mmol Na$^+$/kg per day, in 20% of infants fed a formula providing 1.9 mmolNa$^+$/kg per day, and in 15% of infants receiving preterm breast milk providing on average 2.2 mmolNa$^+$/kg per day during the first 6 weeks of life. This direct relationship between plasma sodium and sodium intake indicates that sodium deficiency rather than water overload is the main cause of *late hyponatraemia* of prematurity.

Sulyok *et al.* (14) have shown in preterm infants (aged 14–42 days) who had low plasma sodium concentrations, that the plasma renin activity and aldosterone concentration rose to high levels at 21 days of age and then declined. This suggests that renal tubular sodium reabsorption is under maximal stimulation at this time, and the evidence shows that in spite of the high aldosterone levels the tubular sodium reabsorption increases more slowly than the glomerular filtration rate during the first weeks of life in preterm infants (14,15,16, 17). The consequent high fractional sodium excretion due to low tubular sodium absorption results initially in negative sodium balance, a contraction of the ECF fluid volume and protective release of antidiuretic hormone. As a result the plasma sodium concentration declines until the filtered sodium matches the tubular sodium reabsorption and a new steady state is reached. More recently Sulyok *et al.* (18) have shown that levels of noradrenalin and dopamine in the urine of breast-fed preterm infants rise to a peak during the 2nd–3rd week after birth, when the plasma sodium was on average 131 mmol/l. Sodium supplements of 3–5 mmol/kg per day both prevented the rise in the urinary catecholamines and resulted in a higher mean plasma sodium concentration of 136 mmol/l.

Maturation of tubular function increases with gestation (16,17,19) and is possibly accelerated by preterm birth (20) and as a consequence the incidence of hyponatraemia diminishes between 32–34 weeks of gestation. French *et al.* (21) showed that infants with a mean gestation of 34 weeks could maintain a normal plasma sodium level whether they were given a full term formula providing 1.2 mmolNa$^+$/kg per day, or a preterm formula providing 3.9 mmolNa$^+$/kg per day. Before this time most preterm infants will need a higher sodium intake per kg body weight than full term infants to maintain a satisfactory plasma sodium concentration (and therefore ECF fluid volume).

There is at present no definition of a satisfactory plasma sodium concentration for preterm infants. We recognize that some infants may apparently tolerate a plasma sodium of less than 130 mmol/l, but for the purpose of these recommendations it is being assumed that the plasma sodium should be maintained above 130 mmol/l (12). From the data on glomerular filtration rate and tubular sodium reabsorption in 2 week old preterm infants published by Sulyok *et al.* (17) it can be calculated that their infants would need an intake of at least 1.8 mmol/kg per day to maintain their plasma sodium concentration at 134 mmol/l in the absence of growth, and since they would require another 1.1 mmol/kg per day for growth it can be inferred that they required at least 2.9 mmol/kg per day for both growth and maintenance of a plasma sodium at 134 mmol/l. However, to raise their plasma sodium to 140 mmol/l it can be calculated that an intake of about 9.0 mmol/kg per day would be required. These estimates show that a relatively modest increase of sodium intake to around 3.0 mmol/kg per day will raise the plasma sodium above 130 mmol/l in most cases, and such an intake corresponds well with the published data (12). In particular intakes of sodium in the region of 3.0 mmol/kg per day have been shown to increase weight gain but without any change in the rate of growth in length or in head circumference (22). However, the large intakes required to achieve a plasma sodium concentration of 140 mmol/l would increase ECF volume and might precipitate heart failure in some infants. They are, therefore, not recommended for routine use.

Insensible sodium losses

There seem to be no measurements of insensible sodium losses in preterm infants but since they sweat very little (23) the losses are likely to be less than those reported in full term infants of 8–12 months which averaged 0.2 mmol/kg per day (24).

Available foods

Sodium in infant formulas

The concentration of sodium in full term formulas available in the United Kingdom ranges from 6.5–13.5 mmol/l which would provide 1.3–2.7 mmol Na^+/kg per day at 200 ml/kg per day. Some formulas designed for low birth weight infants have higher concentrations (providing up to 3.9 mmol Na^+/kg per day), while others provide no more than full term formulas.

Sodium in breast milk

The concentration of sodium in human milk falls during lactation and representative values are given in Table 8.1. A preterm infant receiving his own mother's milk may be expected to ingest the amounts of sodium indicated in Table 8.1 if taking 200 ml/kg per day. Infants receiving formulas designed for full term infants would receive less during the first 3 weeks of life (see above), though they would receive more than that provided by mature human milk which would be about 1.3 mmol/kg per day.

Table 8.1 Sodium concentration of milk of mothers delivering infants of 34 weeks of gestation or less (13).

Week of lactation	Concentration mmol/1	Intake (at 200 ml/kg per day) mmol/kg per day
1.	17.2	3.4
2.	13.7	2.7
3.	12	2.4
4.	9.9	2.0
5.	8.5	1.7
6.	6.5	1.3
7.	8.3	1.7
8.	7.6	1.5
9 & 10	5.7	1.1
11 & 12	6.0	1.2
Pooled mature milk	6.7	1.3

Requirements and advisable intakes

Recommendations of other bodies

ESPGAN Committee on Nutrition (1977): (25) (full term infants). 'The Na Content should not be less than that of human milk but should probably not exceed 1.76 mmol/100 kcal (12 mmol/l)'.

Department of Health and Social Security (1980): (26) (full term infants).
0.65–1.5 mmol/100 ml
0.93–2.2 mmol/100 kcal

American Academy of Pediatrics: Committee on Nutrition (1977) (27). 'Minimum and maximum levels of sodium, chloride, and potassium in formulas for LBW infants (should) be the same as those recommended for full term infants until further work confirms a higher suggested need' (0.9 mmol/100 kcal).

Canadian Paediatric Society Nutrition Committee (1981): (28). 'The total daily sodium requirement in the first weeks of life appears to be 3.0 mmol/100 kcal' '. . . infants weighing less than 1500 g at birth usually require additional sodium, sufficient to raise the total daily sodium intake to 3 mmol/kg until they attain a body weight of 1500 g or a post conceptual age of 34 weeks.'

American Academy of Pediatrics: Committee on Nutrition (1985) (29) (LBW infants). 'Special formulas for premature infants should provide 2.5–3.5 mEq/kg per day at full feeding levels. Very LBW (<1500 g) infants, however, may require 4–8 mEq/kg per day of sodium to prevent hyponatraemia.'

Conclusions

Preterm infants receiving as little as 1.6 mmol/kg per day have been shown to be in positive balance but develop late hyponatraemia (11,12,13). On an intake of 2.3 mmol/kg per day retentions can resemble intrauterine retentions very closely (10) but on this intake some infants will also develop hyponatraemia (13). From calculations based on measurements of renal function and from published data, it can be inferred that an intake between 3.0–5.0 mmolNa$^+$/kg per day would be sufficient for growth, and to maintain the plasma sodium concentration above 130 mmol/l in most infants <1.5 kg with hyponatraemia during the first 4–6 weeks of life (i.e. up to 32–34 weeks of gestation). Between 34 weeks and full term the requirements will fall to about 1.5–2.5 mmol/kg per day. Increasing numbers of babies of birth weight 500–1000 g are surviving and little is known about their renal function. Hyponatraemia is more common in these babies and some of them may require sodium in excess of the amounts recommended here.

We have not recommended that the concentration of sodium in the formula is increased for two reasons.

1 It would still be necessary to supplement many babies, particularly those of VLBW.

2 Since it is not possible to remove sodium from milk some babies may get more sodium than they need, if for example they are more than 32 weeks gestation, or have heart disease.

Guidelines

Breast milk

1 Pooled mature human milk (containing 6.5 mmol Na$^+$/l) even when fed at 200 ml/kg per day may not provide enough sodium for growth and maintenance of plasma sodium concentration over 130 mmol/l in VLBW preterm infants. Therefore the plasma sodium concentration should be closely monitored, and supplements of sodium should be given when required (usually 2–4 mmol/kg per day as sodium chloride).

2 The use of the infant's own mother's milk should reduce the incidence of hyponatraemia because of its higher sodium content.

Formulas

1 For reasons outlined above it is impossible to provide the optimal sodium intake for all preterm infants from a single formula.

2 Because of the possibility of exceeding an infant's sodium requirements as

his renal function matures we do not think that formulas designed for preterm infants should contain more sodium than the upper limit recommended for full term infants (15 mmol/l (27)). We therefore recommend that the sodium concentration of formulas for preterm infants should be similar to that recommended for full term formulas, namely 6.5–15 mmol/l (1.0–2.3 mmol/ 100 kcal), and that the intake should not be less than 1.3 mmol/kg per day.

3 As in the case of breast milk (see p. 109 above) regular monitoring of plasma sodium concentration is required and sodium supplements should be given when necessary.

POTASSIUM

Nutritional background

Potassium is the principal intracellular cation in the body. It contributes to the intracellular osmotic activity and in part determines the intracellular fluid volume. It contributes to the structure and function of proteins, and plays a fundamental part together with sodium in membrane transport, and in the propagation of the nerve and muscle action potential.

Potassium in the fetal body

The potassium concentration in the fetal body remains almost constant during the last trimester of gestation. It is 42.6 mmol/kg at 25 weeks gestation (500 g body weight) and 41.7 mmol/kg at term (3.5 g body weight) (2). The estimated daily rate of accumulation *in utero* lies between 0.6 and 0.8 mmol/kg per day (2,3).

Potassium deficiency

Deficiency is characterized by muscle weakness, paralytic ileus, loss of urinary concentrating ability, hypochloraemic, hypokalaemic alkalosis, and flattening of the T waves of the ECG. In the absence of abnormal losses of potassium from the body, potassium deficiency is unlikely to occur.

Absorption of potassium by preterm infants

Six preterm infants of <1.5 kg birth weight who were fed breast milk with a mean potassium concentration of 15.1 mmol/l received 3.2 mmol/kg per day. They absorbed 2.3 mmol/kg per day and retained 0.9 mmol/kg per day, an amount close to the estimated *in utero* accumulation rate (10).

Available foods

Potassium in infant formulas

The concentration of potassium in full term infant formulas available in the United Kingdom though variable is mostly higher than in human milk and ranges from 14.5–25.5 mmol/l. Formulas designed for preterm infants contain between 19–25 mmol/l.

Potassium in breast milk

The concentration of potassium in human milk is given in Table 8.2. The concentration is highest in early milk and falls throughout lactation. During the second week an infant fed breast milk at 200 ml/kg per day would receive 3.1 mmol of potassium, whereas a formula-fed baby given the same volume would be likely to receive 4.1 mmol/kg per day (range 3.0–5.1 mmol/kg per day).

Table 8.2 Potassium concentration in milk from mothers who have delivered infants of 34 weeks gestation or less (13).

Week of lactation	Concentration mmol/l	Intake (at 200 ml/kg per day) mmol/kg per day
1.	17.5	3.5
2.	15.3	3.1
3.	12.9	2.6
4.	12.9	2.6
5.	12.0	2.4
6.	11.7	2.3
7.	10.0	2.0
8.	10.5	2.1
9 & 10	10.7	2.1
11 & 12	11.3	2.3
Pooled mature milk	10.2	2.0

Requirements and advisable intakes

Recommendations of other bodies

ESPGAN Committee on Nutrition (1977): (25) (full term) 'the sum of sodium, chloride and potassium should not exceed 50 mEq/l'.

Department of Health and Social Security (1980): (26) (full term infants). 13–26 mmol/l of reconstituted feed.

American Academy of Pediatrics: Committee on Nutrition (1977): (27). 'minimum and maximum levels of sodium, chloride and potassium in formulas for low birth weight infants (should) be the same as those recommended for full term infants until further work confirms a higher suggested need.' (2.1 mmol/100 kcal)

Canadian Paediatric Society: Nutrition Committee (1981): (28). No specific recommendation.

American Academy of Pediatrics: Committee on Nutrition (1985): (29) (low birth weight infants). 'The potassium requirement of LBW infants appears to be similar to that of term infants, 2–3 mEq/kg per day.'

Recommendations

Preterm infants do not have problems with potassium homeostasis comparable to those experienced with sodium. The amounts present in breast milk appear satisfactory, as do the rather larger amounts present in formula feeds and should be used as guidelines.

Guidelines

Breast milk

Breast milk with a potassium concentration of 10–17.5 mmol/l (1.5–2.6 mmol/ 100 kcal at 67 kcal/100 ml) contains enough potassium. Fed at 130 kcal/kg per day it provides 2.0–3.5 mmol/kg per day.

Formulas

Formulas with a potassium concentration of 15–25 mmol/l (2.3–3.9 mmol/100 kcal at 65 kcal/100 ml) contain enough potassium. Fed at 130 kcal/kg per day they would provide 3.0–5.0 mmol/kg per day.

CHLORIDE

Nutritional background

Chloride is the principal anion in the ECF compartment and together with sodium contributes more than 80% of the osmotic activity. It is an essential component of membrane transport systems together with sodium and potassium. Though the majority of the body chloride is in the extracellular space some is intracellular (1).

Chloride in the fetus

The chloride concentration in the human fetus falls from 70 mmol/kg at 25 weeks gestation (500 g body weight) to 46 mmol/kg at term (3.5 kg body weight) (1) and accumulates at an average rate of 0.7 mmol/kg per day (3).

Chloride deficiency

Dietary chloride deficiency is rare, but has been described in a group of full term infants receiving a soy based formula with a low concentration of chloride (<1.0–3.0 mmol/l) (30,31), in 30 infants fed an adapted cow's milk formula containing <3.0 mmol Cl^-/l (32) and in two breast-fed full term infants whose mother's milk contained <2.0 mmol Cl^-/l (33,34). The syndrome consisted of failure to thrive, anorexia, muscular weakness, lethargy, vomiting and dehydration. On investigation there was a low plasma chloride, hyponatraemia, hypokalaemia, hypercalcaemia, metabolic alkalosis. Examination of the urine showed low or absent chloride and microscopic haematuria.

Available foods

Chloride in milk

The chloride content of breast milk is given in Table 8.3. The concentration falls in the course of lactation as does that of sodium. Infant formulas designed for full term infants contain 10.5–16.3 mmol/l, and those designed for preterm infants contain 13–23 mmol/l.

Table 8.3 Chloride content of human milk from mothers who have delivered infants of 34 weeks gestation or less (13).

Week of lactation	Concentration mmol/l	Intake (at 200 ml/kg per day) mmol/kg per day
1.	22.1	4.4
2.	18.7	3.7
3.	16.3	3.3
4.	14.5	2.9
5.	11.4	2.3
6.	11.8	2.4
7.	11.6	2.3
8.	12.4	2.5
9 & 10	11.2	2.2
11 & 12	12.3	2.5
Pooled mature milk	12.3	2.5

Requirements of other bodies

Recommendations of other bodies

ESPGAN Committee on Nutrition (1977): (25) (full term infants). 'The sum of the sodium chloride and potassium should not exceed 50 mmol/l.'

Department of Health and Social Security (1980): (26) (full term infants). '11–23 mmol chloride per litre of reconstituted feed.'

American Academy of Pediatrics: Committee on Nutrition (1977): (27) (low birth weight infants). 1.55–4.23 mmol/100 kcal

Canadian Paediatric Society: Nutrition Committee (1981): (28) (low birth weight infants). No comment.

American Academy of Pediatrics: Committee on Nutrition (1985): (29) (low birth weight infants).

800–1200 g (26–28 weeks of gestational age)	3.1 mEq/kg per day
	2.4 mEq/100 kcal
1200–1800 g (29–31 weeks of gestational age)	2.5 mEq/kg per day
	2.0 mEq/100 kcal

Recommendations of this committee

In view of the reported cases of chloride deficiency, low chloride levels in milk must be avoided. The chloride provided by infant formulas (11–16 mmol/l) seems sufficient to prevent chloride deficiency and, provided the breast milk is not chloride deficient, so are the amounts present in breast milk. However, sodium chloride supplements may be necessary in the treatment of sodium depletion (see p. 109).

Guidelines

1   Breast milk with a chloride concentration of 11–22 mmol/l (1.6–3.3 mmol/ 100 kcal at 67 kcal/100 ml) contains enough chloride to prevent chloride deficiency. Fed at 130 ml/kg per day it provides 2.2–4.3 mmol/kg per day.
2   Formulas with a chloride concentration of 11–16 mmol/l (1.6–2.5 mmol/ 100 kcal at 65 kcal/100 ml) also provide enough chloride to prevent chloride deficiency. Fed at 130 kcal/kg per day they would provide 2.1–3.3 mmol/kg per day.
3   If sodium supplements are required they should be given as sodium chloride.

REFERENCES

1. Widdowson E.M. & Dickerson J.W.T. (1961). Chemical composition of the body. In: *Mineral Metabolism*. Vol. 2. (eds C.L. Comer & F. Bronner) Chapter 17. Academic Press, New York.
2. Widdowson E.M. (1982). Importance of nutrition in development with special reference to feeding low birth weight infants. In: *Proc. 2nd Ross. Clin. Res. Conf. Meeting Nutritional Goals for Low birth Weight Infants*. pp. 4–11. Ross Lab, Columbus, Ohio.
3. Shaw J.C.L. (1973). Parenteral nutrition in the management of sick low birth weight infants. *Paediatr. Clin. N. Am.* **20**, 333–58.
4. Lorenz J.M., Kleinman L.I., Kotagal U. & Reller M.D. (1982). Water balance in very low birth weight infants: relationship to water and sodium intake and effect on outcome. *J. Pediatr.* **101**, 423–32.
5. Butterfield J., Lubchenko L., Bergstedt J. & O'Brien D. (1960). Patterns in electrolyte and nitrogen balance in the newborn premature infant. *Pediatrics* **26**, 777–91.
6. Hamilton C.M. & Shaw J.C.L. (1984). Changes in sodium and water balance, renal function and aldosterone excretion during the first seven days of life in very low birth weight infants [Abstract]. *Pediatr. Res.* **18**, 91.
7. Friis-Hansen B. (1961). Body water compartments in children: changes during growth and related changes in body composition. *Pediatrics* **28**, 169–81.
8. Rees L., Brook C.G.D., Shaw J.C.L. & Forsling M.L. (1984). Hyponatraemia in the first week of life in preterm infants. Part I. Arginine vasopressin secretion. *Arch. Dis. Child.* **59**, 414–22.
9. Rees L., Shaw J.C.L., Brook C.G.D. & Forsling M.L. (1984). Hyponatremia in the first week of life in preterm infants. Part II. Sodium and water balance. *Arch. Dis. Child.* **59**, 423–9.
10. Shaw J.C.L. (1982). Absorption and retention of sodium, potassium, magnesium and calcium by preterm infants. In: *Proc. 2nd Ross. Clin. Res. Conf. Meeting Nutritional Goals for Low Birth Weight Infants*. pp. 97–103. Ross Lab, Columbus, Ohio.
11. Day G.M., Radde I.C., Balfe J.W. & Chance G.W. (1976). Electrolyte abnormalities in very low birth weight infants. *Pediatr. Res.* **10**, 522–6.
12. Roy R.N., Chance G.W., Radde I.C., Hill D.E., Willis D.M. & Sheepers J. (1976). Late hyponatraemia in very low birth weight infants (< 1.3 kg). *Pediatr. Res.* **10**, 526–31.
13. Gross S.J. (1983). Growth and biochemical response of preterm infants fed human milk or modified infant formula. *N. Eng. J. Med.* **308**, 237–41.
14. Sulyok E., Németh M., Tenyi I., Csaba I., Györy E., Ertle T. & Varga F. (1979). Postnatal development of Renin-Angiotensin-Aldosterone system, RAAS, in relation to electrolyte balance in premature infants. *Pediatr. Res.* **13**, 817–20.
15. Ross B., Cowett R.M. & Oh W. (1977). Renal functions of low birth weight infants during the first two months of life. *Pediatr. Res.* **11**, 1162–4.
16. Arant B.S. (1978). Developmental patterns of renal functional maturation compared in the human neonate. *J. Pediatr.* **72**, 705–12.
17. Sulyok E., Varga F., Györy E., Jobst K. & Csaba I.F. (1979). Postnatal development of renal sodium handling in premature infants. *J. Pediatr.* **95**, 787–92.
18. Sulyok E., Gyodi G., Ertl T., Bodis J. & Hartmann G. (1985). The influence of NaCl supplementation on the postnatal development of urinary excretion of noradrenalin, dopamine, and serotinin in premature infants. *Pediatr. Res.* **19**, 5–8.
19. Aperia A., Bröberger O., Elinder G., Herin P. & Zetterström R. (1981). Postnatal development of renal function in preterm and fullterm infants. *Acta Paediatr. Scand.* **70**, 183–7.
20. Al-Dahhan J., Haycock G.B., Chantler C. & Stimmler L. (1983). Sodium homeostasis in mature and immature neonates. 1. Renal aspects. *Arch. Dis. Child.* **58**, 335–42.

21. French T.J., Colbeck M., Burman D., Spiedel B.O. & Hendy R.A. (1982). A modified cows milk formula suitable for low birth weight infants. *Arch Dis. Child.* 57, 507-10.
22. Chance G.W., Radde I.C., Willis D.M., Roy R.N., Park E. & Ackerman I. (1977). Postnatal growth of infants of < 1.3 kg birthweight: Effects of metabolic acidosis, of caloric intake, and calcium, sodium and phosphate supplementation. *J. Pediatr.* **91**, 787–93.
23. Harpin V.A. & Rutter N. (1982). Sweating in preterm babies. *J. Pediatr.* **100**, 614–8.
24. Cooke R.E., Pratt E.J. & Darrow D.C. (1950). The metabolic response of infants to heat stress. *Yale J. Biol. Med.* **22**, 227–49.
25. Guidelines on infant nutrition. (1977). 1. Recommendations for the composition of an adapted formula. *Acta Paediatr. Scand.* (Suppl.) 262.
26. Department of Health and Social Security. Report No. 18. (1980). *Artificial Feed for the Young Infant.* HMSO, London.
27. American Academy of Pediatrics Committee on Nutrition (1977). Nutritional needs of low birth weight infants. *Pediatrics* **60**, 519–30.
28. Canadian Paediatric Society Nutrition Committee (1981). Feeding the low birth weight infant. *Can. Med. Ass. J.* 301–11.
29. American Academy of Pediatrics: Committee on Nutrition (1985). Nutritional needs of low birthweight infants. *Pediatrics* **75**, 976–86.
30. Roy A. III & Arant B.S. (1979). Alkalosis from Chloride deficient Neo-Mul-Soy. *N. Eng. J. Med.* **301**, 615.
31. Grossman H., Duggan E., McCamman S., Welchert E. & Hellerstein S. (1980). Dietary chloride deficiency syndrome. *Pediatrics* **66**, 366–74.
32. Rodrigues-Sorriano J., Vallo A., Castillo G., Oliveros R., Cea J.M. & Balzategui M.J. (1983). Biochemical features of dietary chloride deficiency syndrome: A comparative study of 30 cases. *J. Pediatr.* **103**, 209–14.
33. Ashes R.S., Wisotsky D.H., Migel P.F., Siegle R.L. & Levy J. (1982). The dietary chloride deficiency syndrome occurring in a breast fed infant. *J. Pediatr.* **100**, 923–4.
34. Hill I.D. & Bowie M.D. (1983). Chloride deficiency syndrome due to chloride-deficient breast milk. *Arch. Dis. Child.* **58**, 224–6.

9
Calcium, Phosphorus and Magnesium

NUTRITIONAL BACKGROUND

Intrauterine accumulation rate

Fetal skeleton acquires 80% of its calcium, magnesium, and phosphorus in the last trimester of gestation. The 1.0 kg fetus contains about 5.7 g of calcium, 3.4 g of phosphorus, and 0.2 g of magnesium. In a 3.5 kg fetus, these values reach 28.8, 16.8 and 0.8 g, respectively (1). In the full term baby, the Ca:P ratio in the body is about 1.7 at birth and 99% of the calcium, 80% of the phosphorus and 65% of the magnesium are in bones (2).

Postnatal accumulation rate

From the chemical analysis of human fetal bodies, it can be calculated that, between 26 and 36 weeks of gestation, the mean accumulation of calcium, phosphorus, and magnesium is about 130, 75 and 3.5 mg per kilo body weight per day, respectively (3,4). Human milk and most standard infant formula do not contain enough calcium and phosphorus to allow preterm infants to accumulate these elements at the intrauterine rate, even if all the calcium and phosphorus were absorbed and retained (5–7).

In artificially fed preterm infants, the net absorption of calcium may be negative soon after birth and it increases with age (8). Calcium absorption may further be affected by a number of factors such as: lactose intake (9), quantity and quality of fat in the diet (10–16), the absolute intakes of calcium and phosphorus and the ratio of these intakes (5,15–24), the presence of phytate (25), intestinal secretion and faecal loss of endogenous calcium (26–30), gestational and postnatal ages (8,19,21,23), and vitamin D status (16–20).

A number of investigators have shown that net calcium absorption and net calcium retention in low birth weight (LBW) infants are related to calcium intake. Preterm infants retain more calcium per unit of body weight with higher calcium intake, even though the percent calcium absorption declines with increasing calcium intake (5,8,12–25).

Metabolic balance studies carried out in preterm infants fed banked *human milk* or their own mother's milk show that net intestinal absorption of calcium is in the range of 50–80% whereas that of phosphorus is about 90% (8,16,22–24). Urinary excretion of phosphorus is negligible but that of calcium is not, being often greater than 10 mg/kg per day (16,19–24). As a result, preterm infants fed human milk retain only 20–25 mg of calcium and phosphorus per kg body weight per day, which corresponds to 15–20% of the calcium and 30–35% of the phosphorus accumulated by the fetus *in utero* (8,16,19–24). Magnesium absorption ranges from 1 to 74% with a mean value of 43% of intake and magnesium retention ranges from 1 to 5 mg/kg per day, i.e. 30–160% of the fetal deposition (19,24,31).

Mineral content of most *infant formulas* is higher than that of human milk. The percentage of absorption of calcium, however, is generally lower so that the amount of calcium retained is not necessarily much higher than with human milk (5,8,12,16,17,19–25,32). Unlike calcium, phosphorus is always well absorbed, net absorption ranging from at least 80% up to 94% (5,16,19–24,32). Lower phosphorus absorption rates have, however, been observed in preterm infants fed soya based formulas (25). In formula-fed infants, in contrast to breast-fed infants, urinary excretion of calcium is usually low whereas that of phosphorus is high (16,19–24,32). Because of the poor calcium absorption, the good absorption of phosphorus and the low glomerular filtration rate, babies receiving unmodified cow's milk formulas may develop hyperphosphataemia causing hypocalcaemia (33–35). Supplementation of infant formulas with calcium salts is generally associated with increased calcium retention (5,17–19). However, this improvement may be overestimated. For example, it has been claimed that oral calcium supplements, as calcium lactate, can result in calcium retention similar in the intrauterine rate (5). There has, however, been some concern (7,16) with the interpretation of these balance data since the phosphate retention was not affected to the same extent by calcium supplementation (5,18) and the apparent calcium:phosphorus retention ratio may be as high as 5:1 (5). This strongly suggests that sedimentation of calcium lactate had occurred in the bottle so that the babies received less calcium than was thought. Magnesium intake is higher from infant formulas than from human milk, but as for calcium there are greater faecal magnesium losses in formula fed preterm infants so that average absorption rates are similar. It has been reported that magnesium retention in preterm infants fed fortified human milk or infant formulas is similar or exceeds the intrauterine retention rate (19,24).

More recently, *preterm infant formulas* have been designed to approach the requirements of LBW infants as estimated by the factorial method (6). As a consequence they usually contain greater amounts of minerals than standard infant formulas, and also well absorbed fat such as medium-chain triglycerides (36). Balance studies with these formulas have demonstrated increased calcium and phosphorus retention. Retentions of minerals as high as or exceeding intrauterine accretion rate were reported (15,37), but as discussed above, these results may be erroneously high in view of the very heavy precipitation of calcium and phosphorus in some of these formula (7,16,38). Sequential measurements of bone mineral density have also demonstrated better bone mineralization in preterm infants fed formulas supplemented with calcium and phosphorus (39). Therefore, though the retention of calcium may not be as high as sometimes claimed, an increase in calcium and phosphorus intake results in a worthwhile improvement in retention of these elements.

Signs of deficiency

Early neonatal hypocalcaemia is commonly found but is mostly asymptomatic in preterm infants (35). There is an appropriate physiologic response of the parathyroid glands to hypocalcaemia; abrupt arrest of maternal calcium supply at birth and, possibly, rapid increase of plasma calcitonin level are the main aetiological factors (35,40–47). Early milk feeding and calcium supplementation by oral (48–50) or intravenous route (42,43,47,51) have been shown to reduce the incidence of hypocalcaemia during the first 72 hours after birth. *Late neonatal hypocalcaemia* occurs generally between 3 and 15 days of age. It may follow early neonatal hypocalcaemia and is often accompanied by seizures. Late enamel hypoplasia of the teeth has also been described (52). Late neonatal hypocalcaemia is more frequently observed during winter and spring in infants with a poor vitamin D status who are fed high phosphate and low calcium:phosphorus ratio formulas (34,35). In these infants, parathyroid response is insufficient to maintain normal plasma calcium and phosphorus concentrations (45). Feeding human milk or infant formulas with reduced phosphorus content, and early administration of vitamin D are prophylactic measures (33–35,45,53,54).

A *phosphorus depletion syndrome* characterized by hypophosphataemia, hypercalciuria, absent urinary phosphorus, signs of bone demineralization, and high serum levels of alkaline phosphatase has been reported in preterm infants fed human milk (16,20–24,55–64) or on total parenteral nutrition with an unbalanced calcium–phosphorus intake (65,66). In full term babies the low phosphorus intake from breast milk is sufficient to meet the requirements of growth although even in those babies the addition of phosphorus has been shown to improve calcium and phosphorus retention (67). In preterm infants, the low intake of phosphorus cannot meet the demand of rapid skeletal and soft tissue growth and so hypophosphataemia occurs more commonly. Resolution of rickets and correction of hypercalciuria, with resultant increase in calcium retention and bone mineral content has been observed in preterm infants fed human milk who were supplemented with phosphate alone (20,57,58,60–62) or with both calcium and phosphorus (59,63,64). Phosphorus content of cow's milk based infant formulas is always higher than that of breast milk. Even when the calcium:phosphorus ratio in the formula has been set at 2 as in human milk, the amount of phosphorus in the formula is such that no case of phosphate depletion syndrome or phosphorus-deficient rickets has been reported in preterm infants fed standard formulas, except when addition of calcium leads to a calcium:phosphorus ratio in intakes higher than 2.0 (63).

Magnesium deficiency is exceptional in healthy neonates. It is essentially associated with maternal magnesium deficiency (35,67). Although low serum magnesium levels may occur in the first 72 hours after birth, the levels rapidly rise to normal adult values within a few days in preterm as well as in full term infants once feeding of either formula or human milk is begun (19,35, 41,47,67). Late hypomagnesaemia has been reported in association with hypocalcaemia; both being corrected by magnesium supplementation (34). It has been shown that magnesium retention is lower (19,31) and that less magnesium is laid down in the bone of preterm infants fed human milk than in the bone of the fetus (68) but nothing comparable is known about magnesium in the soft tissues.

Hypomineralization of bone (commonly called osteopenia) or signs of overt rickets have been reported in preterm infants fed in various ways: human milk (7,8,19–24,55–63,69,70), soy formulas (25,71,72), standard proprietary infant formulas (5,8,19,71,73–75) and total parenteral nutrition (65,66,76). Incidence of rickets as high as 50% has been reported in VLBW preterm infants (77). In some patients this has been associated with fractures (72,78) and respiratory distress (79). Diagnosis of inadequate bone mineralization have been based on different criteria: radiological observations (5,19,21,60, 61,69,72,73,80,81); mineral balance studies (7,8,12,16,17,19–32); biochemical values (19–24,57,63,70–72,77,82–86); post-mortem analysis of bone structure (73,76) and mineral composition (68,87). A significant correlation has been found between raised plasma alkaline phosphatase activity and radiological changes so that determination of plasma alkaline phosphatase levels could be of value in screening for rickets in preterm infants (82,84–86). Markedly increased plasma alkaline phosphatase values have, however, been observed in preterm infants both in the presence and absence of clinical and radiological signs of rickets (21,24). Recently, serial measurements of radial bone mineral density by direct photon absorptiometry has been utilized for monitoring bone mineralization in preterm infants (39, 59,75,88,89). Using this technique, it appeared that bone mineralization in preterm infants fed human milk or a standard infant formula lagged significantly behind that achieved *in utero* (75,90). However, the reliability of the method has been questioned (91). The pathogenesis of skeletal lesions in preterm infants is usually multifactorial. Inadequate calcium and/or phosphorus intakes are the main factor (5,7,19–30,55–94), calcium mal-absorption (8,12,16,17,28–30), inadequate vitamin D intake or metabolism (16,20,41,53,72,74,79–83,92,93), copper deficiency (see section on copper), increased acid load (81), and chronic diuretic therapy (95) have also been implicated. Calcium supplementation of infant formulas (5,19,63,89,93) and calcium as well as phosphorus supplementation of human milk (19–24,57–62, 69–79) have been shown to improve signs of bone mineralization in VLBW infants. Using photon absorptiometry, it has been claimed that preterm infants fed formulas supplemented with calcium and phosphorus have improved bone mineralization during the first 3 months of life (39,90). While delayed bone mineralization of preterm infants is related to inadequate intakes of calcium and phosphorus, the role of vitamin D metabolites on the regulation of calcium and phosphorus absorption and their direct and indirect effects on skeletal development can not be ignored. This is discussed in the section on vitamin D (Chapter 7, p. 71).

AVAILABLE FOODS

Human milk

Mature human milk contains 25–34 mg of calcium, 11–16 mg of phosphorus, and 3–4 mg of magnesium per dl, and the calcium:phosphorus ratio ranges from 1.8 to 2.2 (96,97). These figures do not differ materially in milk from mothers of preterm infants (19,98–101).

Human milk routinely supplemented with phosphorus alone or with both calcium and phosphorus has been used for feeding of preterm infants. The addition of 9 mg of phosphorus/dl from solution of disodium or dipotassium phosphate has been shown to be sufficient to correct the phosphate depletion syndrome (16,20,23,57–62,64). Simultaneous addition of calcium and phosphate salts result in immediate precipitation of calcium phosphates. If, however, phosphate is first mixed with human milk and then calcium is added, the solution is much more stable. In these conditions, addition of calcium gluconate, up to 70 mg of calcium per dl, and of disodium phosphate, up to 50 mg of phosphorus per dl, is stable over-night (64).

Infant formulas

Mineral content of cow's milk based infant formulas varies over a wide range. Calcium and phosphorus being partly linked to casein (102), the content of these minerals is generally related to protein content and whey:casein ratio in the formula. However, in some formulas with a high whey:casein ratio, calcium, phosphorus, and magnesium salts are added by the manufacturers. The lowest calcium, phosphorus, and magnesium contents are 60, 30 and 6 mg/100 kcal, respectively, although in several currently available infant formulas values twice as high or more are found. The calcium:phosphorus ratio in infant formulas varies from 1.1 to 2.2 according to the recommendations of different bodies (105,113).

Low birth weight infant formulas

Formulas specially designed for LBW infants generally contain more minerals than conventional infant formulas. Certain formulas developed in the United States contain up to 180 mg of calcium, 90 mg of phosphorus and 19 mg of magnesium per 100 kcal (36), but it should be noted that precipitation of calcium and phosphate salts has occurred in some of these formulas (38). LBW infant formulas presently available in Europe contain less minerals: 70–140 mg of calcium and 40–80 mg of phosphorus per 100 kcal but even in these some precipitation may occur.

REQUIREMENTS AND ADVISABLE LIMITS

The ideal postnatal rate of bone mineralization in preterm infants is unknown. Although it may not be necessary (7), it has been recommended for the nutritional management of these infants that protein and minerals are provided in amounts which will allow accretion of nutrients at rates similar to those occurring *in utero* during the third trimester of gestation (5,6,103,104). Employing a factorial method, Ziegler *et al.* (6) summed the tissue accretion of nutrients with estimates of urinary and dermal losses and, allowing for imperfect absorption, derived theoretical mineral requirements for infants of varying gestational ages. Advisable intakes per kg body weight per day as high as 210 mg of calcium, 140 mg of phosphorus and 10 mg of magnesium have been proposed for 1000 g preterm infants, these figures becoming 185, 123 and 8.5 mg/kg per day, respectively, for 1500 g infants (6). It is obvious that mineral content of human milk and most infant formulas cannot meet these calculated requirements, but calcium and phosphate can be added and several studies have shown an improvement of mineral retention, and/or bone mineralization in preterm infants receiving higher calcium and phosphorus intakes than those supplied by human milk or most infant formulas (5,15–24,37,39, 57–64,93). Whether it is necessary to accumulate minerals at the same rate as the fetus is, however, questionable. Indeed, decreasing density and remodelling of bone occur in term infants after birth and may be a physiologic event (2). The very high concentrations of minerals in some formulas are not without risk to preterm infants. For example, too high an intake of phosphorus may lead to hyperphosphataemia which blocks the production of 1,25-di-hydroxy-vitamin D and results in hypocalcaemia (106); too high an intake of calcium has been associated with fat bolus obstruction and lacto-bezoar formation in the gastrointestinal tract (107,108); high calcium intake may impede fat absorption (5,16,109); and high calcium retention may induce metabolic acidosis since calcification of the skeleton is a source of net acid (11). For these reasons we believe that very high calcium and phosphorus intakes based on the factorial method of calculation should not be administered to VLBW infants. Indeed, there is evidence that preterm infants fed formulas containing 80 mg/dl (120 mg/100 kcal) of calcium do not develop bone disease and have normal plasma activity of alkaline phosphatases (86). Moreover it has been shown that bone mineral content in preterm infants at age 4–16 years is appropriate for the size of children (11).

In contrast to calcium which is mainly deposited in bones, phosphorus is required for new tissue synthesis as well as for bone mineralization. Phosphorus accumulation is related to nitrogen and calcium retentions following the equation:

$$P \text{ retention (in mg)} = Ca \text{ retention}/2.2 + N \text{ retention}/15.$$

This equation clearly shows that optimal calcium:phosphorus ratio in the milk cannot be constant. Indeed, assuming that nitrogen retention per kg body weight in preterm infants is 300–350 mg/kg per day, as in the fetus, phosphorus accumulation in new tissues will be about 20 mg/kg per day. If calcium intake is low, for example 70 mg/kg per day with an absorption rate of 70%, 49 mg of calcium/kg per day can be deposited in bones together with an addition of 24 mg of phosphorus. In these conditions assuming an absorption rate of 90% total phosphorus intake must be at least 50 mg/kg per day, i.e. a calcium:phosphorus ratio of 1.4/1.0. On the other hand, if calcium intake is high, for example 160 mg/kg per day with an absorption rate of 50%, 80 mg of calcium can be deposited in bones together with 36 mg of phosphorus. In these conditions, a total phosphorus intake of 80 mg/kg per day is sufficient, i.e. a calcium:phosphorus ratio in milk of 2/1. Thus because of the high nitrogen retention of VLBW infants, the lower the calcium intake, the lower must be the calcium:phosphorus ratio in the milk to meet the phosphorus requirements but if calcium content of the milk is high, the calcium:phosphorus ratio should be higher.

Advisable intake in a preterm infant fed human milk

Phosphorus

As noticed above (see Nutritional background) in rapidly growing preterm infants fed human milk, particularly in those less than 1300 g, the very low phosphorus intake may lead to a typical phosphate-depletion syndrome with hypophosphataemia, hypophosphaturia, hypercalciuria, rickets, and elevated plasma alkaline phosphatase activity. Resolution of rickets and hypercalciuria, with resultant increase in calcium retention and bone mineral content, have been reported with phosphate supplementations. A plasma inorganic concentration below 4.6 mg/dl or 1.5 mmol/l together with either a urinary excretion of calcium greater than 6 mg/kg per day or a urinary calcium:phosphorus ratio (in mg) higher than one are good indicators of the need for phosphorus supplementation. Phosphorus may be added to breast milk (see available food) or may be given as a supplement to correct bone lesions or routinely to prevent the phosphorus deficiency in growing preterm infants.

Calcium

Addition of calcium salts or protein without phosphate supplementation in human milk must be avoided in growing preterm infants since it aggravates the phosphorus-depletion syndrome and may lead to very high urinary excretion of calcium with risk of nephrocalcinosis (112). On the other hand, supplementation of human milk with calcium and phosphorus salts (see available food) has been shown to improve calcium and phosphorus retention and bone mineral density in preterm infants.

Magnesium

Human milk contains about 3 mg of magnesium per dl and no biochemical signs of magnesium deficiency have been reported in healthy preterm infants fed breast milk. Although some babies receiving breast milk retain magnesium below the *in utero* accumulation rate and have slightly lower serum magnesium concentration than formula-fed babies, frank hypomagnesaemia is rare and we do not recommend the addition of magnesium routinely to breast milk.

Vitamin D

Human milk contains less vitamin D activity than previously thought and vitamin D supplementation is needed (see Chapter 7).

Advisable intake in preterm infant fed formulas

Lower limits

Preterm infants fed standard full term infant formulas rarely develop bone disease, provided vitamin D status is adequate. However, VLBW infants will probably benefit from greater mineral intakes, since their requirements in calcium and phosphorus are higher than those of full term infants per unit body weight until they have completed rapid 'catch-up' growth and attained a metabolic maturity similar to that of their full term counterpart.

Therefore the minimum mineral content of preterm infant formulas should be a little higher than the recommended minimum content in standard infant formulas, i.e. 60 mg of calcium and 30 mg of phosphorus per 100 kcal (112). In fact, the mineral content usually found in infant formulas is about 70 mg of calcium, 50 mg of phosphorus, 6 mg of magnesium per 100 kcal and may be adopted as a lower limit.

Upper limits

Calcium salts added to infant formulas are poorly soluble and may precipitate. Calcium losses approaching 50% have been observed in high mineral content preterm infant formulas when the formula is delivered continuously by a pump during a 4 hour period (117). Because of the possible complications of very high calcium intake, the problem of precipitation, and the lack of evidence that such high concentrations are beneficial, the upper limit of calcium intake should not exceed 140 mg/100 kcal.

Phosphorus is much better absorbed than calcium and too high an intake of phosphorus may lead to hyperphosphaturia, hyperphophataemia and hypo-calcaemia (see Nutritional background). Since phosphorus accumulation is related to nitrogen and calcium deposition (see p. 125) and assuming that net calcium absorption will be 75% at most, the provision of 90 mg of phosphorus per 100 kcal will not result in phosphorus deficiency, when the calcium intake is 140 mg/100 kcal, and will minimize the risk of phosphorus overload. This concentration is therefore a reasonable upper limit to adopt.

Calcium:phosphorus ratio: the optimum ratio in a formula cannot be constant because of the need of phosphorus for new tissue synthesis and a Ca:P ratio of 2.2 in bones. As indicated on p. 125, the Ca:P ratio in milk must be reduced when calcium concentration is low, and it should be increased when calcium content is high. Therefore, the calcium:phosphorus ratio in the preterm infant formulas may suitably range from 1.4 to 2.0 according to the calcium content.

Magnesium deficiency or overload has not been reported in preterm infants fed standard infant formulas. Preterm infants fed fortified human milk or preterm formula containing 5.4 and 8.6 mg of magnesium per 100 kcal, respectively, had a magnesium retention similar to or higher than the estimate of fetal accretion (24). Owing to the possible interaction with absorption and excretion of other divalent anions, there is no evidence that the magnesium content in preterm formulas should exceed 12 mg/100 kcal.

These recommendations should be followed in conjunction with those for vitamin D (see Chapter 7, p. 71).

GUIDELINES

Breast milk

In VLBW infants at risk of developing phosphate depletion syndrome and bone disease, phosphate supplementation is suggested up to 13 mg/100 kcal (i.e. 17 mg/kg per day at 130 kcal/kg per day) either alone or added to the milk. There is evidence to recommend calcium supplementation.

If this is done, calcium supplements alone should not be given without a proportionate amount of phosphate in order to maintain the calcium: phosphate ratio in the range of 1.4–2.0. In any case we see no reason for exceeding the maximal calcium intake achieved with proprietary formulas (i.e. 140 mg/100 kcal). There is not sufficient evidence to recommend magnesium supplementation of human milk.

Infant formulas

Calcium: minimum 70 mg/100 kcal (1.75 mmol/100 kcal)
             maximum 140 mg/100 kcal (3.5 mmol/100 kcal)
Phosphorus: minimum 50 mg/100 kcal (1.6 mmol/100 kcal)
             maximum 90 mg/100 kcal (2.9 mmol/100 kcal)
Magnesium: minimum 6 mg/100 kcal (0.25 mmol/100 kcal)
             maximum 12 mg/100 kcal (0.5 mmol/100 kcal)
Ca/P: minimum 1.4:1.0
             maximum 2.0:1.0

REFERENCES

1. Widdowson E.M. & Dickerson J.W.T. (1964). Chemical composition of the body. In: *Mineral Metabolism* Vol. 2A. (eds C.L. Comar & F. Bronner) pp 1–247. Academic Press, New York.
2. Royer P. (1981). Growth and development of bony tissue. In: *Scientific Foundations of Paediatrics.* (eds J.A. Davis & J. Dobbing) pp 565–90. William Heinemann Medical Books Ltd, London.

3. Shaw J.C.L. (1973). Parenteral nutrition in the management of the sick low birthweight infant. *Pediatr. Clin. N. Am.* **20**, 333–58.

4. Forbes G.B. (1976). Calcium accumulation by the human fetus. *Pediatrics* **57**, 976–7.

5. Day G.M., Chance G.W., Radde I.C., Reilly B.J., Park E. & Sheepers J. (1975). Growth and mineral metabolism in very low birthweight infants. II. Effects of calcium supplementation on growth and divalent cations. *Pediatr. Res.* **9**, 568–75.

6. Ziegler E.E., Biga R.L. & Fomon S.J. (1981). Nutritional requirements of premature infants. In: *Pediatric Nutrition.* (ed. R.M. Suskind) pp 29–39. Raven Press, New York.

7. Atkinson S.A. (1983). Calcium and phosphorus requirements of low birth weight infants: a nutritional and endocrinological perspective. *Nutr. Rev.* **41**, 69–78.

8. Shaw J.C.L. (1976). Evidence for defective skeletal mineralization in low birthweight infants. The absorption of calcium and fat. *Pediatrics* **57**, 16–25.

9. Ziegler E.E. & Fomon S.J. (1983). Lactose enhances mineral absorption in infancy. *J. Pediatr. Gastroenterol. Nutr.* **2**, 288–94.

10. Southgate D.A.T., Widdowson E.M., Smits B.J., Cooke W.T., Walker C.H.M. & Mathers N.P. (1969). Absorption and excretion of calcium and fat by young infants. *Lancet* **1**, 487–9.

11. Williams M.L., Rose C.S., Morrow G. III, Sloan S.E. & Barness L.A. (1970). Calcium and fat absorption in neonatal period. *Am. J. Clin. Nutr.* **23**, 1322–30.

12. Barltrop D. & Oppé T.E. (1973). Absorption of fat and calcium by low birthweight infants from milks containing butterfat and olive oil. *Arch. Dis. Child.* **48**, 496–501.

13. Roy C.C., Ste-Marie M., Chartrand L., Weber A., Bard H. & Doray B. (1975). Correction of the malabsorption of the preterm infant with a medium-chain triglyceride formula. *J. Pediatr.* **86**, 446–50.

14. Tantibhedhyangkul P. & Hashim S.A. (1978). Medium-chain triglyceride feeding in premature infants: Effects on calcium and magnesium absorption. *Pediatrics* **61**, 537–45.

15. Shenai J.P., Reynolds J.W. & Babson S.G. (1980). Nutritional balance studies in very-low-birth weight infants: Enhanced nutrient retention rates by an experimental formula. *Pediatrics* **66**, 233–8.

16. Senterre J. & Salle B. (1982). Calcium and phosphorus economy of the preterm infant and its interaction with vitamin D and its metabolites. *Acta Paediatr. Scand.* (Suppl.) **296**, 85–92.

17. Barltrop D. & Oppé T.E. (1973). Calcium and fat absorption by low birthweight infants from a calcium-supplemented milk formula. *Arch. Dis. Child.* **48**, 580–2.

18. Moya M. & Domenech E. (1982). Role of calcium-phosphate ratio of milk formulae on calcium balance in low birthweight infants during the first three days of life. *Pediatr. Res.* **16**, 675–80.

19. Atkinson S.A., Radde I.C. & Anderson G.H. (1983). Micromineral balances in premature infants fed their own mothers' milk or formula. *J. Pediatr.* **102**, 99–106.

20. Senterre J., Putet G., Salle B. & Rigo J. (1983). Effects of vitamin D and phosphorus supplementation on calcium retention in preterm infants fed banked human milk. *J. Pediatr.* **103**, 305–7.

21. Lyon A.J. & McIntosh N. (1984). Calcium and phosphorus balance in extremely low birth weight infants in the first six weeks of life. *Arch. Dis. Child.* **59**, 1145–50.

22. Rowe J., Rowe D., Horak E. *et al.* (1984). Hypophosphatemia and hypercalciuria in small premature infants fed human milk: Evidence for inadequate dietary phosphorus. *J. Pediatr.* **104**, 112–17.

23. Carey D.E., Goetz C.A., Horak E. & Rowe J.C. (1985). Phosphorus wasting during phosphorus supplementation of human milk feedings in preterm infants. *J. Pediatr.* **107**, 790–7.

24. Schanler R.J., Garza C. & O'Brian Smith E. (1985). Fortified mothers' milk for very low birth weight infants: Results of macromineral balance studies. *J. Pediatr.* **107**, 767–74.

25. Shenai J.P., Jhaveri B.M., Reynolds J.W., Huston R.K. & Babson S.G. (1981). Nutritional balance studies in very-low-birth-weight infants: Role of soy formula. *Pediatrics* **67**, 631–7.

26. Sutton A. & Barltrop D. (1973). Absorption, accretion and endogenous faecal excretion of calcium by the newborn infant. *Nature* **242**, 265.

27. Senterre J. (1976). Endogenous faecal calcium, total digestive juice calcium, net and true calcium absorption in premature infants. In: *Perinatal Medicine, Prague, August 1974.* (eds Z.K. Stembera, K. Polacek & V. Sabata) pp. 287—8 George Thieme, Stuttgart.

28. Barltrop D., Mole R.H. & Sutton A. (1977). Absorption and endogenous faecal excretion of calcium by low birthweight infants on feeds with varying contents of calcium and phosphate. *Arch. Dis. Child.* **52**, 41–9.

29. Ehrenkranz K.A., Ackermans B.A., Nelli C.M. & Janghorbani M. (1985). Absorption of calcium in premature infants as measured with a stable isotope ^{46}Ca extrinsic tag. *Pediatr. Res.* **19**, 178–84.

30. Moore L.J., Machlan L.A., Lim M.O., Yergey A.L. & Hansen J.W. (1985). Dynamics of calcium metabolism in infancy and childhood. I: Methodology and quantification in the infant. *Pediatr. Res.* **19**, 329–34.

31. Dauncey M.J., Shaw J.C.L. & Urman J. (1977). The absorption and retention of magnesium, zinc, and copper by low birthweight infants fed pasteurized human breast milk. *Pediatr. Res.* **11**, 991–7.

32. Senterre J. & Lambrechts A. (1972). Nitrogen, fat and mineral balances in premature infants fed acidified or non acidified half-skimmed cow milk. *Biol. Neonate* **20**, 107–19.

33. Oppé T.E. & Redstone D. (1968). Calcium and phosphorus levels in healthy newborn infants given various types of milk. *Lancet* **1**, 1045–6.

34. Cockburn F., Brown J.K., Belton N.R. & Forfar J.O. (1973). Neonatal convulsions associated with primary disturbance of calcium, phosphorus and magnesium metabolism. *Arch. Dis. Child.* **48**, 99–108.

35. Tsang R.C., Donovan E.F. & Steichen J.J. (1976). Calcium physiology and pathology in the neonate. *Pediatr. Clin. N. Am.* **23**, 611–26.

36. Brady M.S., Rickard K.A., Ernst J.A., Schreiner P.L. & Lemons J.A. (1982). Formulas and human milk for premature infants: A review and up date. *J. Am. Diet. Ass.* **81**, 547–55.

37. Gibbs J.A.H. (1982). Early and late growth effects of increased mineral and whey protein intake by tiny infants. In: *Proceedings of the Second Ross Clinical Research Conference: Meeting Nutritional Goals for Low-Birth-Weight Infants.* pp 29–37. Ross Laboratories, Colombus Ohio.

38. Bhatia J. & Fomon S.J. (1983). Formulas for premature infants: fate of the calcium and phosphorus. *Pediatrics* **72**, 37–40.

39. Greer F.R., Steichen J.J. & Tsang R.C. (1982). Effects of increased calcium, phosphorus, and vitamin D intake on bone mineralization in very low-birth-weight infants fed formulas with polycose and medium-chain triglycerides. *J. Pediatr.* **106**, 951–5.

40. David L., Salle B., Chopard P. & Grafmeyer D. (1977). Studies on circulating immunoreactive calcitonin in low birthweight infants during the first 48 hours of life. *Helv. Paediatr. Acta* **32**, 39–48.

41. Hillman L.S., Rojanasathit S., Slatopolsky E. & Haddad J.G. (1977). Serial measurements of serum calcium, magnesium, parathyroid hormone, calcitonin and 25-hydroxy-vitamin D in premature and term infants during the first week of life. *Pediatr. Res.* **11**, 739–44.

42. Salle B.L., David L., Chopard J.P., Grafmeyer D.C. & Renaud H. (1977). Prevention of early neonatal hypocalcemia in low birth weight infants with continuous calcium infusion: effect on serum calcium, phosphorus, magnesium and circulating immunoreactive parathyroid hormone and calcitonin. *Pediatr. Res.* **11**, 1180–5.

43. David L., Salle B., Putet G. & Grafmeyer D. (1981). Serum immunoreactive calcitonin in low birthweight infants. Description of early changes; effect of intravenous calcium infusion; calcium, phosphorus, magnesium, parathyroid hormone and gastrin levels. *Pediatr. Res.* **15**, 803–8.

44. Salle B.L., David L., Glorieux F.M., Delvin E., Senterre J. & Renaud H. (1982). Early oral

administration of vitamin D and its metabolites in premature neonates. Effect on mineral homeostasis. *Pediatr. Res.* **16**, 75–8.

45. David L., Glorieux F.M., Salle B.L. & Anast C.S. (1983). Human neonatal hypocalcemia. In *Calcium and Phosphorus Metabolism* (eds M.F. Holick, T.K. Gray & C.S. Anast) pp 351–61. Elsevier Science Publishers, Amsterdam.
46. Scott S.M., Ladenson J.H., Aquanna J.J., Walgate J. & Hillman L.S. (1984). Effect of calcium therapy in the sick premature infant with early neonatal hypocalcemia. *J. Pediatr.* **104**, 747–51.
47. Cooper L.J. & Anast C.S. (1985). Circulatory immunoreactive parathyroid hormone levels in premature infants and the response to calcium therapy. *Acta Paediatr. Scand.* **74**, 669–73.
48. Brown D.R., Tsang R.C. & Chen I.W. (1976). Oral calcium supplementation in premature and asphyxiated neonates. *J. Pediatr.* **89**, 973–7.
49. Moya M. & Domenech E. (1978). Calcium intake in the first five days of life in the low birthweight infant. Effects of calcium supplements. *Arch Dis. Child.* **53**, 714–17.
50. Sann L., David L., Chayvialle J.A. *et al.* (1980). Effect of early oral calcium supplementation on serum calcium and immunoreactive calcitonin concentration in preterm infants. *Arch Dis. Child.* **55**, 611–15.
51. Brown D.R., Steranka B.H. & Taylor F.H. (1981). Treatment of early-onset neonatal hypocalcaemia. Effects on serum calcium and ionized calcium. *Am. J. Dis. Child.* **135**, 24–8.
52. Mellander M., Noren J.G., Freden H. & Kjellmer I. (1982). Mineralization defects in deciduous teeth of low birthweight infants. *Acta Paediatr. Scand.* **71**, 727–33.
53. Glorieux F.K., Salle B.L., Delvin E.E. & David L. (1981). Vitamin D metabolism in preterm infants: serum calcitriol values during the first five days of life. *J. Pediatr.* **99**, 640–43.
54. Salle B., David L., Glorieux C., Delvin E.E., Louis I.J. & Troney G. (1982). Hypocalcemia in infants of diabetic mothers. *Acta Paediatr. Scand.* **71**, 573–7.
55. Yllpö A. (1919). Das Wachstum der Frügeborenen von der Geburt bis zum Schulalter. *Z. Kinderheilk.* **24**, 111–22.
56. Von Sydow G. (1946). A study of the development of rickets in premature infants. *Acta Paediatr. Scand.* (Suppl. II) **33**, 1–22.
57. Rowe J.C., Wood D.H., Rowe D.W. & Reisz L.G. (1979). Nutritional hypophosphatemic rickets in a premature infant fed breast milk. *N. Engl. J. Med.* **300**, 293–950.
58. Sagy M., Birenbaum E., Balin A., Orda S., Barzilay Z. & Brish M. (1980). Phosphate-depletion syndrome in a premature infant fed human milk. *J. Pediatr.* **96**, 683–5.
59. Greer F.R., Steichen J.J. & Tsang R.C. (1982). Calcium and phosphate supplements in breast milk-related rickets. Results in a very-low-birth-weight infant. *Am. J. Dis. Child.* **136**, 581–3.
60. Koo W.W.K., Gupta J.H., Nayanar V.V., Wilkinson M. & Posen S. (1984). Continuous nasogastric phosphorus infusion in hypophosphatemic rickets of prematurity. *Am. J. Dis. Child.* **138**, 172–5.
61. Lyon A.J., McIntosh N., Wheeler K. & Brooke O.G. (1984). Hypercalcaemia in extremely low birth weight infants. *Arch. Dis. Child.* **59**, 1171–7.
62. Sann L., Loras B., David L. *et al.* (1985). Effect of phosphate supplementation to breast fed very low birth weight infants on urinary calcium excretion, serum immunoreactive parathyroid hormone and plasma 1.25 dihydroxy-vitamin D concentration. *Acta Paediatr. Scand.* **74**, 664–8.
63. Laing I.A., Glass E.J., Hendry G.M.A. *et al.* (1985). Rickets of prematurity: Calcium and phosphorus supplementation. *J. Pediatr.* **106**, 265–8.
64. Salle B., Senterre J., Putet G. & Rigo J. (1986). Effects of calcium and phosphorus supplementation on calcium retention and fat absorption in preterm/pooled infants fed human milk. *J. Pediatr. Gastroenterol Nutr.* **5**, 638—42.
65. Leape L.L. & Valaes T. (1976). Rickets in low birth weight infants receiving total parenteral nutrition. *J. Pediatr. Surg.* **11**, 665.

66. Chessex P., Pincault M., Zebiehe H. & Ayotte R.A. (1985). Calciuria in parenterally fed preterm infants: role of phosphorus intake. *J. Pediatr.* **107**, 794–6.
67. Widdowson E.M., McCance R.A., Harrison G.E. & Sutton A. (1963). Effect of giving phosphate supplements to breast fed babies on absorption and excretion of calcium, strontium, magnesium and phosphorus. *Lancet* **ii**, 1250.
68. McIntosh N., Shaw J.C.L. & Taghizadeh A. (1974). Direct evidence for calcium and trace mineral deficits in the skeleton of preterm infants. *Pediatr. Res.* **8**, 896.
69. Kooh S.W., Fraser D., Reilly B.J., Hamilton J.R., Gall D.G. & Bell L. (1977). Rickets due to calcium deficiency. *N. Engl. J. Med.* **297**, 1264–6.
70. Koo W.W.K., Gupta J.M., Nayanar V.V., Wilkinson M. & Posen S. (1982). Skeletal changes in preterm infants. *Arch Dis. Child.* **57**, 447–52.
71. Hoff N., Haddad J., Teitelbaum S., McAlister W. & Hillman L.S. (1979). Serum concentrations of 25-hydroxyvitamin D in rickets of extremely premature infants. *J. Pediatr.* **94**, 460–6.
72. Kulkarni P.B., Hall R.T., Rhodes P.G. *et al.* (1980). Rickets in very low-birthweight infants. *J. Pediatr.* **96**, 249–52.
73. Griscom W.T., Craig J.N. & Neuhauser R.B.D. (1971). Systemic bone disease developing in small premature infants. *Pediatrics* **48**, 883–93.
74. Lewin P.K., Reid M., Reilly B.J., Swyer P.P. & Fraser D. (1971). Iatrogenic rickets in low birthweight infants. *J. Pediatr.* **78**, 207–10.
75. Minton S.D., Steichen J.J. & Tsang R.C. (1979). Bone mineral content in term and preterm appropriate for gestational-age infants. *J. Pediatr.* **95**, 1037–42.
76. Pfenheimer S.J. & Snodgrass G.J.A.I. (1980). Neonatal rickets. Histopathology and quantitative bone changes. *Arch Dis. Child.* **55**, 945–9.
77. McIntosh N., Livesey A. & Brooke O.G. (1982). Plasma 25-hydroxyvitamin D and rickets in infants of extremely low birthweight. *Arch. Dis. Child.* **57**, 848–50.
78. Geggel R.L., Pereira G.R. & Spackman T.J. (1978). Fractured ribs: Unusual presentation of rickets in premature infants. *J. Pediatr.* **93**, 680–82.
79. Glasgow J.F.T. & Thomas P.S. (1977). Rachitic respiratory distress in small preterm infants. *Arch. Dis. Child.* **52**, 268–73.
80. Bosley A.R.J., Verrier E.R. & Campbell M.J. (1980). Aetiological factors in rickets of prematurity. *Arch. Dis. Child.* **55**, 683–6.
81. Radde I.C., Chance G.W., Bailey K., O'Brien J., Day G.M. & Sheepers J. (1973). Effects of correction of late metabolic acidosis on growth and minerals in very low birthweight (< 1.3 kg) infants. *Pediatr. Res.* **7**, 170.
82. Kovar I., Mayne P. & Barltrop D. (1982). Plasma alkaline phosphatase activity: a screening test for rickets in preterm neonates. *Lancet* **i**, 308–10.
83. Kovar I.Z., Mayne P. & Wallis J. (1982). Neonatal rickets in one of identical twins. *Arch. Dis. Child.* **57**, 792–4.
84. Kovar I. & Mayne P. (1981). Plasma alkaline phosphatase activity in the preterm neonate. *Acta Paediatr. Scand.* **70**, 501–6.
85. Glass E.J., Hume R., Hendry G.M.A., Strange R.C. & Forfar J.O. (1982). Plasma alkaline phosphatase activity in rickets of prematurity. *Arch. Dis. Child.* **57**, 373–6.
86. Gross S.J. (1983). Growth and biochemical response of preterm infants fed human milk or modified infant formula. *N. Engl. J. Med.* **308**, 237–41.
87. Shaw J.C.L. (1982). Absorption and retention of sodium, potassium, magnesium, and calcium by preterm infants. In: *Proceedings of the Second Ross Clinical Research Conference: Meeting Nutritional Goals for Low-Birth-Weight Infants*. pp. 97—103.Ross Laboratories, Colombus Ohio.
88. Minton S.D., Steichen J.J. & Tsang R.C. (1983). Decreased bone mineral content in small-for-gestational-age infants compared with appropriate-for-gestational-age infants: normal serum 25-hydroxyvitamin D and decreasing parathyroid hormone. *Pediatrics* **71**, 383–8.

89 Steichen J.J., Tsang R.C., Greer F.R., Ho M. & Hug G. (1981). Elevated serum 1,25 dihydroxyvitamin D concentrations in rickets of very low-birth-weight infants. *J. Pediatr.* **99**, 293–8.

90. Steichen J.J., Gratton T.L. & Tsang R.C. (1980). Osteopenia of prematurity: the cause and possible treatment. *J. Pediatr.* **96**, 528–34.

91. Tyson J.E., Maravilla A., Lasky R.E., Cope F.A. & Mize C.E. (1983). Measurement of bone mineral content of preterm neonates. Reliability of the Norland densitometer. *Am. J. Dis. Child.* **137**, 735–7.

92. Callenbach J.C., Sheehan M.B., Abramson S.J. & Hall R.T. (1981). Etiologic factors in rickets of very low-birth-weight infants. *J. Pediatr.* **98**, 800–5.

93. Cifuentes R.F., Kooh S.W. & Radde I.C. (1980). Vitamin D deficiency in a calcium supplemented very low-birth-weight infant. *J. Pediatr.* **96**, 252–5.

94. Lapatsanis P., Makaronis G., Vretos C. & Doxiadis S. (1976). Two types of nutritional rickets in infants. *Am. J. Clin. Nutr.* **29**, 1222–6.

95. Hufnagle K.G., Khan S.N., Penn D., Cacciarelli A. & Williams P. (1982). Renal calcification: a complication of long term furosemide therapy in preterm infants. *Pediatrics* **70**, 360–3.

96. Barltrop D. & Hillier R. (1974). Calcium and phosphorus content of transitional and mature human milk. *Acta Paediatr. Scand.* **63**, 347–50.

97. Feeley R.M., Eitenmiller R.R., Jones J.B. & Barnhart H. (1983). Calcium, phosphorus, and magnesium contents of human milk during early lactation. *J. Pediatr. Gastroenterol. Nutr.* **2**, 262–70.

98. Gross S.J., David R.J., Bauman L. & Tomarelli R.M. (1980). Nutritional composition of milk produced by mothers delivering pre-term. *J. Pediatr.* **96**, 641–4.

99. Atkinson S.A., Radde I.C., Chance G.W. *et al.* (1980). Macro-mineral content of milk obtained during early lactation from mothers of premature infants. *Early Hum. Dev.* **4**, 5–140.

100. Sann L., Bienvenu J., Bienvenu F., Lahet C. & Bethenod M. (1981). Comparison of the composition of breast milk from mothers of term and preterm infants. *Acta Paediatr. Scand.* **70**, 115–60.

101. Chan G.M. (1982). Human milk calcium and phosphate levels of mothers delivering term and preterm infants. *J. Pediatr. Gastroenterol. Nutr.* **1**, 201–5.

102. Fransson G.B. & Lonnerdal B. (1983). Distribution of trace elements and minerals in human and cows milk. *Pediatr. Res.* **17**, 412–15.

103. American Academy of Pediatrics, Committee on Nutrition (1977). Nutritional needs of low birth weight infants. *Pediatrics* **60**, 519.

104. Canadian Paediatric Society, Nutrition Committee (1981). Feeding the low birth weight infant. *Can. Med. Ass. J.* **124**, 1301.

105. Department of Health and Social Security (1980). *Artificial Feeds for the Young Infant.* Report on Health and Social Subjects No. 18. pp 42–5. HMSO, London.

106. Deluca H.F. (1980). Some new concepts emanating from a study of the metabolism and function of vitamin D. *Nutr. Rev.* **38**, 169.

107. Brooke O.G., Gentner P.R., Harzer G. & Spitz L. (1982). Milk fat bolus obstruction in a preterm infant. *Acta Paediatr. Scand.* **71**, 691.

108. Schreiner R.L., Lemons J.A. & Gresham E.L. (1979). A new complication of nutritional management of the low birth weight infant. *Pediatrics* **63**, 683.

109. Katz L. & Hamilton J.R. (1974). Fat absorption in infants of birth weight less than 1300 g. *J. Pediatr.* **85**, 608.

110. Kildeberg P., Engel K. & Winters R.W. (1969). Balance of net acid in growing infants. Endogenous and transintestinal aspects. *Acta Paediatr. Scand.* **58**, 321.

111. Helin I., Landin L.A. & Nilsson B.E. (1985). Bone mineral content in preterm infants at age 4 to 16. *Acta Paediatr. Scand.* **74**, 264–7.

112. Goldsmith M.A., Bhatia S.S., Kanto U.P., Kutner M.H. & Rusman D. (1981)Gluconate calcium therapy and neonatal hypercalciuria. *Am. J. Dis. Child.* **135**, 538–43.
113. ESPGAN Committee on Nutrition (1977). Guidelines on infant nutrition I: Recommendations for the composition of an adapted formula. *Acta Paediatr. Scand.* (Suppl.) **262**.
114. Antonson D.L., Smith J.L. & Welson R.D. (1983). Stability of vitamin concentrations of low birth weight infant formula during continuous enteral feeding. *J. Pediatr. Gastroenterol Nutr.* **2**, 617–21.

10
Iron

NUTRITIONAL BACKGROUND

Iron in the fetal body

A 1.0 kg fetus contains about 64 mg Fe (1). Between 24 and 36 weeks of gestation iron in the fetal body increases at approximately 1.8 mg Fe/kg per day (2) and fetuses weighing over 3.0 kg have been shown to contain 90 ± 25 mg/kg iron (1). The distribution of the iron in the body is not known for certain — in the adult about 70% is in haemoglobin, 5% is myoglobin and 15% is in the ferritin iron stores while a small proportion (about 0.1%) is in the haem and non-haem enzymes (3). However, measurements of non-haem iron in fetal livers (4) indicate that a larger proportion — about 25% of the body iron of a 1.0 kg infant is present as ferritin iron stores. Since the amount of iron in a 1.0 kg infant is sufficient to synthesize only 18.0 of haemoglobin, such babies will become iron deficient by the time they double their birth weight if fed on milks such as breast milk which have a low iron content (vide infra).

Anaemias of prematurity

Early anaemia

Following birth there is a rise in PaO_2 and a fall in the secretion rate of erythropoietin (5,6). This results in a decline in the bone marrow activity and a fall in haemoglobin concentration to a plateau of around 9.0 g/100 ml between 4 and 6 weeks of age. Iron liberated at this time enters the iron stores. Between 4 and 6 weeks of age there is a reticulocytosis and a more active haematopoiesis is resumed, the haemoglobin mass increases but the haemoglobin concentration remains constant because of growth, or may fall a little if the volume of distribution enlarges faster than the haemoglobin mass.

Late anaemia

If iron intake is inadequate, iron stores will become exhausted between 6 and 8 weeks in infants <1400 g and between 8 and 12 weeks in those >1400 g (7) and judging from serum ferritin levels significant iron deficiency occurs in some infants of 1–2 kg birth weight from about 8 weeks onwards (8). When iron stores are exhausted the haemoglobin mass cannot increase, and the haemoglobin concentration will fall, resulting in late anaemia. Iron administration will prevent or cure the late anaemia but has no effect on the early anaemia (7).

From these considerations it is evident that iron is not an essential component of the diet immediately after birth, but must be supplied in sufficient amounts before the iron stores become depleted.

Iron absorption

Iron once present in the body cannot be excreted in any significant amount, so in health the amount of iron in the body is determined by a process of controlled absorption (9,10). Iron in the intestine is bound to a variety of ligands of which one is lactoferrin. There is initial binding of iron to specific receptors on the microvillus membrane (11), it is then transported from the mucosal to the serosal pole of the enterocyte bound to a transport protein that has been identified as a transferrin (12,13,14). There is evidence that a part of the process is energy dependent suggesting that iron absorption is effected by active carrier mediated transport (15). Ferritin, also present in the enterocyte, probably plays a secondary, though important role in safely binding iron that enters the enterocyte but which is not to be absorbed.

The mechanism by which the body communicates its need for iron to the mucosal cell is at present unknown. Though erythropoietin does not itself augment iron absorption, stimuli that increase erythropoiesis (such as anaemia or a low PaO_2) tend to increase iron absorption, and conversely stimuli that inhibit erythropoiesis (such as hypertransfusion or an elevation of PaO_2) inhibit iron absorption (16,17,18,19,20).

This brief review is based mainly on studies on adult man and animals and little is known about the development of control of iron absorption in the fetus or preterm infant.

AVAILABLE FOODS

Iron in breast milk

The concentrations of iron in breast milk at different periods of lactation are given in the Table 10.1. There is no difference in its concentration in the milk of mothers of full term infants and in the milk of mothers of preterm infants. It appears that the concentration of iron in breast milk declines slightly during the course of lactation (21,22) but not everyone has observed this change (23). The concentration of iron in pooled breast milk is in the region of 40 μg/100 ml (23). About 30% of the iron in milk is associated with the lipid fraction, and 36% is bound to unidentified low molecular weight proteins of <15000 (23). Lactoferrin (M_r 75000) is the principal iron binding protein in milk (3.3±1.9 g/l) (23) and though it contains 24% of the iron in human milk, it is only 1.4% saturated. This very high unsaturated iron binding capacity enables lactoferrin to inhibit bacterial growth by complexing free iron (24,25). It should be noted, however, that lactoferrin is also found in bile, pancreatic and intestinal secretions. It coats the luminal surface of the intestine and may have the additional function of binding dietary iron prior to donating it to surface receptors on the duodenal brush border (26).

Table 10.1. Comparison of the changes of iron concentration in milk from mothers of full term and preterm infants (21).

Postnatal age	Full term μg/100 ml ±s.d.		Preterm μg/100 ml ±s.d.	
3–5 days	111	±43	110	±34
8–10 days	99	±31	99	±27
12–17 days	81	±20	93	±41
28–30 days	88	±28	90	±23

Iron in formulas

The iron concentrations in some infant formulas are given in Table 10.2. Some have added iron (generally in the form of ferrous fumarate) and others do not. The amount added to most full term formulas aims to provide between 1.0–2.0 mg/kg per day at an intake of 150 ml/kg per day. In the USA formulas are available with, and without added iron. For example, one LBW formula (81 kcal/100 ml) without added iron contains 0.2 mg iron/100 ml while the same formula with iron contains 1.46 mg iron/100 ml (29). The formula with added iron would therefore provide just over 2.0 mg iron/kg per day when fed at 120 kcal/kg per day (150 ml/kg per day).

Table 10.2. Iron concentration of different infant formulas

Country of origin	No of samples	Iron µg/100 ml Mean	Range	Reference
USA	14	2.8	0.02–5.90	(27)
Sweden	12	0.33	0.08–1.20	(27)
West Germany	12	0.37	0.01–1.30	(27)
Japan	8	0.77	0.56–1.30	(27)
The Netherlands	2	0.35	0.20–0.50	(27)
England	2	0.60	0.43–0.76	(27)
Full term formula	9	0.77	0.71–0.86	(28)
Preterm formula	3	0.81	0.72–0.95	(28)
Soy formula	1	1.38		(28)
France	2	0.57	0.55–0.90	(27)
Norway	1	0.90		(27)

Bioavailability

There are now a number of investigations that all tend to indicate that iron added to breast milk is better absorbed than iron added to either cow's milk (30) or to formulas (31). It is not clear to what extent this is due to different bioavailability or to the intestinal blood loss associated with cow's milk based feeds (32). Whatever the cause, the effect has not been shown to be large enough to warrant increasing the concentration of iron in formula feeds for full term infants. Indeed there has been a recent trend to reduce the concentration of iron in formulas to 0.6–0.7 mg/100 ml. This has resulted in part from studies of iron absorption in full term infants (30,33), but also from fears of increasing the risk of bacterial infections (24), and of inducing lipid peroxidation of red cell membranes and haemolysis (34). The induction of bacterial infections by giving too much iron is a potentially serious risk but has only been documented following the use of parenteral iron dextran (35,36). The risk of causing significant haemolysis on the other hand seems to be very small if vitamin E intake is sufficient (7,37,38).

Iron balance of preterm Infants

Absorption

Preterm infants who are given unsupplemented human breast milk with an iron content of about 40 µg/100 ml are in negative iron balance of the order of –0.2 mg/kg per day for at least one month after birth (39) and in some cases for as long as 4–5 months after birth (40). Full term small for gestational age infants by contrast may be in positive iron balance (39). Increasing iron intake increases iron absorption in both full term (30) and premature infants (39). In full term infants the percentage iron absorption falls with increasing iron intake (30) indicating a measure of control over iron absorption, but in preterm infants this seems not to be the case. Measurements of iron absorption in preterm infants suggest that it is a linear function of iron intake, and dependent upon the concentration in the diet rather than the amount of iron in the body (39). Therefore, if given too little iron they will absorb insufficient, and if given too much they may absorb too much and be at risk from iron overload. There is much evidence to indicate that an intake of 2.0–2.5 mg/kg per day is sufficient for haemoglobin synthesis and prevents the late anaemia of prematurity (7,39,41). Siimes *et al.* (1982) (42) have given up to 4.0 mg/kg per day to VLBW infants. Though this higher dose prevents the late anaemia of prematurity it has not been shown to be better than the lower dose, and may be associated with abnormal elevations of the plasma ferritin (43) (vide infra).

Factors modifying iron requirements

Losses of iron from the body

On very low iron intakes, endogenous loss of iron by the intestine can be significant and is estimated to be about 0.21 mg/kg per day, and an intake of about 0.6 mg/kg per day would be required to compensate for these losses and maintain zero net absorption (43). Iron in the urine is generally undetectable. Insensible iron losses from the skin and hair have not been measured in preterm infants and can only be estimated from measurements in adults (44). Scaled down on the basis of surface area the losses would appear to be small — in the order of 0.02 mg/kg per day. Losses from blood sampling are potentially much greater, since each gram of haemoglobin contains 3.4 mg of iron.

Gains of iron by the body

The administration of iron by blood transfusion can be substantial. In 12 infants of <1500 g birth weight receiving between 3 and 8 transfusions, the iron given was approximately 55 ± 17 mg (mean$\pm$s.d.) and corresponded to an average retention of 1.5 mg/day (45). Though transfusion may depress iron absorption the effect is transient and the degree of depression depends on the size of the transfusion, so some iron is absorbed in spite of the transfusion (39). Measurement of serum ferritin in preterm infants (gestation $\pm$ s.d, 28 ± 1.3 wks, birth weight$\pm$s.d., 1098 ± 149 g) who received 3–8 blood transfusions and iron supplements of 5.0 mg/kg per day are consistent with a moderate though transient period of iron overload in about half the infants (43). Though no morbidity was observed in these infants and the ferritin levels declined spontaneously when transfusions were stopped, the results do indicate that infants (generally the smallest and most immature) who are given regular top up transfusions do not need simultaneous iron supplements.

REQUIREMENTS
AND ADVISABLE INTAKES

Recommendations of Other Bodies

ESPGAN Committee on Nutrition: (46) (full term infants). 'Iron: 0.1–0.2 mg/100 kcal (0.07–0.14 mg/100 ml) (formulas without iron supplementation). Not less than 1.0 mg/100 kcal (0.7 mg/100 ml) (formulas with iron supplementation).'

Department of Health and Social Security: (47) (full term infants). '. . .a reconstituted infant feed should contain not less than 70 μg iron/100 ml and not more than 700 μg/100 ml.'

American Academy of Pediatrics (1976): (41). 'In breast fed infants. . . the dose of supplemental iron should not exceed. . . 2.0 mg/kg per day for preterm infants, up to a maximum of 15 mg/kg per day (as supplemental iron drops of ferrous sulphate). For formula fed infants an iron supplemented formula is recommended (10–12 mg/l as ferrous sulphate).

American Academy of Pediatrics: (1977) (48). '. . . though the committee. . . continues to recommend that low birth weight infants receive 2.0 mg of iron per kilogram per day starting at age 2 months or earlier, one cannot categorically require that formulas provide this level of iron from birth. . . formulas for low birth weight infants may provide either 0.1 mg or 1.5 mg of iron per 100 kcal.'

Canadian Paediatric Society: Nutrition Committee (1981) (49). Breast-fed preterm infants: 2.0 mg/kg per day.
'Formulas used for the low birth weight infants provide between 0.1 and 1.5 mg of iron per 100 kcal.'

American Academy of Pediatrics: Committee on Nutrition (1978) (50) (low birth weight infants). 'Infants fed human milk should be fed 2–3 mg/kg per day of elemental iron as ferrous sulphate drops; formulas with iron usually contain sufficient supplemental iron. A somewhat higher total daily dose of iron (supplemental plus iron in formula) has been recommended by Siimes: this regimen should be started by the age of 2 months and continued to the age of 12–15 months.'

Iron requirements

From the evidence reviewed above and from the results of the deliberations of other bodies it is probable that most if not all late iron deficiency of prematurity can be prevented by giving 2.0–2.5 mg Fe/kg per day (to maximum of 15 mg/day), starting not later than 2 months of age and continuing throughout the remainder of the first year of life. We see no reason to differ, in the main, from these recommendations (41,47,48,49,50) but think they require some amplification.

There are increasing numbers of infants of <1.0 kg birth weight surviving today and yet very little is known about their ability to control the absorption of dietary iron. Since blood transfusions are commonly given to these small preterm infants to maintain haemoglobin levels, their iron stores may be preserved or augmented to the extent that the iron given in transfusions, equals or exceeds that lost by blood sampling and via the intestine. It is therefore *unlikely* that the iron stores of regularly transfused infants will be exhausted by 6–8 weeks of age as they would be, if no transfusions or iron supplements were given. Since dietary iron may be a factor in the aetiology of gram negative infections in preterm infants it would seem reasonable to give a milk, like breast milk, that contains no added iron during the first 6–8 weeks of life. Such formulas are available in the USA (29). However, many formulas designed for preterm infants do contain added iron, and to date no harm from their use has been reported, even though they have been given from the initiation of oral feeding. This iron is absorbed (39) and will prevent a transitory iron deficiency in some infants whose iron stores might otherwise become exhausted before iron supplements were introduced (41).

With the data presently available we cannot make a firm recommendation on whether or not it is desirable to feed an iron free formula during the first eight weeks of life, particularly in those infants of less than 1.0 kg birth weight. Variations in management in individual cases, such as the number of blood tests and transfusions, will have a bearing on iron requirements. If, however, it is the practice to maintain the haemoglobin concentration with regular blood transfusions then iron supplements are not required until the regular transfusions are stopped.

There are virtually no data indicating how long iron supplements should be continued after discharge home. It would seem prudent to maintain them until full mixed feeding is established.

GUIDELINES

1 Infants fed breast milk or formulas with no added iron should be

supplemented with 2.0–2.5 mg Fe/kg per day from not later than 8 weeks of age (maximum 15 mg Fe/day).

2 Infants who are fed formula with added iron should be supplemented if necessary with sufficient iron to achieve a total iron intake of 2.0–2.5 mg Fe/kg per day from not later than 8 weeks of age (maximum 15 mg Fe/day).

3 A formula aiming to provide all iron requirements should contain approximately 1.5 mg Fe/100 kcal which in the energy range 110–165 kcal/kg per day would provide 1.7–2.5 mg/kg per day of iron. At an energy density range of 65–85 kcal/100 ml the concentration would be 0.98–1.28 mg/100 ml.

4 Infants receiving regular blood transfusions to maintain their haemoglobin concentration: delay the introduction of oral iron supplements until transfusions have ceased.

5 On discharge home: fully breast-fed infants should receive 2.0 mg/kg per day to a maximum of 15 mg/day. Formula fed infants receiving an iron fortified formula probably receive sufficient iron.

6 Iron supplements should be continued until full mixed feeding providing an adequate iron intake is established (usually 12–15 months).

REFERENCES

1. Widdowson E.M. & Dickerson J.W.T. (1969). *Chemical Composition of the Body. Mineral Metabolism.* Vol 2. Part A. (eds C.L. Comar & F. Bronner) Academic Press, New York.
2. Shaw J.C.L. (1973). Parenteral nutrition in sick low birthweight infants. *Pediatr. Clin. N. Am.* **20**, 333–58.
3. Underwood E.J. (1971). *Trace Elements in Human and Animal Nutrition.* 3rd edn. Academic Press, New York.
4. Chang L.L. (1972). Storage iron in fetal livers. *Acta Paediatr. Scand.* **62**, 173–5.
5. Halvorsen S. & Finne P.H. (1968). Erythropietin production in the human fetus and the newborn. *Ann. N. Y. Acad. Sci.* **149**, 576–7.
6. Halvorsen S. (1963). Erythopoietin levels in cord blood and in blood during the first weeks of life. *Acta Paediatr.* **53**, 425.
7. Seip M. & Halvorsen S. (1956). Erythrocyte production and iron stores in premature infants during the first months of life: The anaemia of prematurity — etiology, pathogenesis, iron requirements. *Acta Paediatr. Scan.* **45**, 600–17.
8. Lundström U., Siimes M.A. & Dallman P.R. (1977). At what age does iron supplementation become necessary in low birth weight infants? *J. Pediatr.* **91**, 878–83.
9. McCance R.A. & Widdowson E.M. (1937). Absorption and excretion of iron. *Lancet* ii, 680–4.
10. McCance R.A. & Widdowson E.M. (1938). The absorption and excretion of iron after oral and intravenous administration. *J. Physiol.* **94**, 148–54.
11. Cox T.M. & O'Donnel M.W. (1981). Iron binding and the transport of iron across the rabbit intestinal brush border. *Biochem. Soc. Trans.* **9**, 157–8.
12. Forth W. & Rummel W. (1973). Iron absorption. *Physiol. Rev.* **53**, 724–92.
13. El-Shobaki F.A. & Rummel W. (1977). Mucosal transferrin and ferritin, factors in the regulation of iron absorption. *Res. Exp. Med.* **171**, 243–53.
14. Savin M.A. & Cook J.D. (1980). Mucosal iron transport by rat intestine. *Blood* **56**, 1029–52.
15. Cox T.M. & Peters T.J. (1979). The kinetics of iron uptake *in vitro* by the duodenal mucosa.

Studies in normal subjects. *J. Physiol.* **289**, 469–78.

16. Reynafarge C. & Ramos J. (1961). Influence of altitude on intestinal iron absorption. *J. Lab. Clin. Med.* **57**, 848–55.

17. Weintraub L.R., Conrad M.E. & Crosby W.H. (1965). Regulation of intestinal absorption of iron by the rat of erythropoiesis. *Br. J. Haematol.* **11**, 432–8.

18. Hathorn M.K.S. (1968). The influence of decompressioned hypoxia on iron absorption and distribution in the rat. Unpublished PhD Thesis. Faculty of Medicine, University of London.

19. Wheby M.S., Jones L.G. & Crosby W.H. (1964). Studies on iron absorption. Intestinal regulatory mechanisms. *J. Clin. Invest.* **43**, 1433–42.

20. Mendel G.A. (1961). Studies on iron absorption. I. The relationship between the rate of erythropoiesis, hypoxia, and iron absorption. *Blood* **18**, 727–36.

21. Mendelson R.A., Anderson G.H. & Bryan M.H. (1982). Zinc, copper and iron content of milk from mothers of preterm infants. *Early Hum. Dev.* **6**, 145–51.

22. Siimes M.A., Vuori E. & Kuitunen P. (1979). Breast milk iron a declining concentration during the course of lactation. *Acta Paediatr. Scand.* **68**, 29–31.

23. Fransson G-B. & Lönnerdal B. (1980). Iron in human milk. *J. Paediatr.* **96**, 380–4.

24. Bullen J.J., Rogers H.J. & Leigh L. (1972). Iron binding proteins in milk and resistance to Escherichia Coli infections in infants. *Br. Med. J.* **1**, 69–75.

25. Bezkorovainy A. (1981). Antimicrobial properties of iron binding proteins. *Adv. Exp. Med. Biol.* **135**, 139–54.

26. Cox T.M., Mazurier J., Spik G., Montreuil J. & Peters T.J. (1979). Iron binding proteins and influx of iron across the dodenal brush border. *Biochem. Biophys. Acta* **588**, 120–8.

27. Lönnderdal B., Keen C.L., Ohtake M. & Tamura T. (1983). Iron, zinc, copper, and manganese in infant formulas. *Am. J. Dis. Child.* **137**,433–7.

28. Shaw J.C.L. Unpublished data.

29. Proc 2nd Ross Clin Res Conf. (1982). *Meeting the Nutritional Goals for Low Birth Weight Infants.* Ross Laboratories, Columbus, Ohio.

30. Saarinen U.M., Siimes M.A. & Dallman P.R. (1977). Iron absorption in infants. High bio-availability of breast milk iron as indicated by extrinsic tag method of iron absorption and by concentration of serum ferritin. *J. Pediatr.* **91**, 36–9.

31. Jarvenpaa A-L., Raîha N.C.R., Gaull G.E. & Siimes M.A. (in prep). Human milk is better than formula for iron nutrition in preterm infants.

32. Fomon S.J., Zeigler E.E., Nelson S.E. & Edwards B.B. (1981). Cow milk feeding in infancy: gastrointestinal blood loss and iron nutritional status. *J. Pediatr.* **98**, 540–5.

33. Saarinen U.M. & Siimes M.A. (1977). Iron absorption from infant milk formula and optimal level of iron. *Acta Paediatr. Scan.* **66**, 719–22.

34. Williams M., Shott R.J., O'Neal P.L. & Oski F.A. (1975). Dietary iron and fat in vitamin E deficiency anaemia of infancy. *N. Engl. J. Med.* **292**, 887–90.

35. Barry D.M.J. & Reeve A.W. (1977). Increased incidence of gram negative neonatal sepsis with intramuscular iron administration. *Pediatrics* **60**, 908–12.

36. Becroft D.M.O., Dix M.R. & Farmer K. (1977). Intramuscular iron-dextran and susceptibility of neonates to bacterial infections. *Arch Dis. Child.* **52**, 778–81.

37. Jansson J., Holmberg J. & Ekman R. (1979). Medicinal iron to low birth weight infants. *Acta Paediatr. Scand.* **68**, 705–8.

38. Rudolf N., Preis O., Bitzos E., Reale M. & Wong S.L. (1981). Hematologic and selenium status of low birth weight infants fed formulas with and without iron. *J. Pediatr.* **99**, 57–62.

39. Dauncey M.J., Davies C.G., Shaw J.C.L. & Urman J. (1978). The effect of iron supplements and blood transfusion on iron absorption by low birth weight infants fed pasteurised human breast milk. *Pediatr. Res.* **58**, 889–904.

40. Lichtenstcin A. (1921). Der Eisenumsatz bei Fruhgeborenen. *Acta Paediatr.* (Uppsala) **1**, 194–239.

41. American Academy of Pediatrics: Committee on Nutrition (1976). Iron Supplement for infants *Paediatrics* **58**, 756–67.
42. Siimes M.A. & Jarvenpaa A-L. (1982). Prevention of anaemia and iron deficiency in very low birth weight infants. *J. Pediatr.* **101**, 277–80.
43. Shaw J.C.L. (1982). Iron absorption by the preterm infant. The effect of transfusion and iron supplements on serum ferritin levels. *Acta Paediatr. Scand.* (Suppl.) **299**, 83–9.
44. Jacob R.A., Sandstead H.H., Munozo J.M., Klevay L.M. & Milne D.B. (1981). Whole body surface loss of trace metals in normal males. *Am. J. Clin. Nutr.* **34**, 1379–83.
45. Shaw J.C.L. Unpublished data.
46. ESPGAN Committee on Nutrition: Guidelines on Infant Nutrition (1977). I Recommendation for the Composition of an Adapted Formula. *Acta Paediatr. Scand.* (Suppl.) **262**.
47. Department of Health and Social Security (1980). *Artificial Feeds for the Young Infant.* Report on Health and Social Subjects. No. 18. HMSO, London.
48. American Academy of Pediatrics: Committee on Nutrition (1977). Nutritional needs of low birth weight infants. *Pediatrics* **60**, 519–30.
49. Canadian Paediatric Society: Committee on Nutrition (1981). Feeding the low birth weight infant. *Can. Med. Ass.* **124**, 1301–11.
50. American Academy of Pediatrics: Committee on Nutrition (1985). Nutritional needs of low birth weight infants *Pediatrics* **75**, 976–86.

11
Zinc

NUTRITIONAL BACKGROUND

In 1934 Todd *et al.* (1) demonstrated that zinc was an essential nutrient in mammals. At the present time more than seventy zinc proteins have been identified — most of them enzymes. Since zinc is a necessary component of both DNA and RNA polymerases it is intimately concerned in the replication, transcription and repair of DNA during cell division and therefore plays a fundamental role in growth (2).

Zinc deficiency

The features of human zinc deficiency are those of acrodermatitis enteropathica which is due to an autosomal recessively inherited defect in zinc absorption (3,4). It is characterized by growth arrest, irritability, anorexia, alopecia, perioral and perineal dermatitis, vesicopustular lesions of the hands and feet, oesophagitis, diarrhoea, thymic atrophy and defects in cell mediated immunity. Experimental zinc deficiency during pregnancy in the rat produces small litters of severely growth retarded pups with a high incidence of congenital malformations (5). There is some evidence that zinc deficiency may also produce malformations in man (6,7).

Zinc in the
fetal body

The concentration of zinc in the fetal body is about 19 ± 5 mg/kg fat free body weight (8). It accumulates at about 249 μg/kg per day during the last trimester of pregnancy (2) and a full term infant contains about 66 mg of zinc (8). At term about a quarter of the body zinc is in the liver in a concentration of 18 mg/100 g wet weight (9) where it is bound to metallothionein (10). About 40% of the body zinc is thought to be present in the skeleton (2), and may prove an important reserve, which can be released as the bones undergo remodelling after birth.

Zinc in milk

Breast milk

The concentration of zinc in breast milk is given in the Tables 11.1 and 11.2. The concentration is very high in colostrum but falls tenfold during the course of lactation (Table 11.1). It is evident that the provision of zinc from colostrum and early milk exceeds the *in utero* accumulation rate if given at a volume of 200 ml/kg per day, but late milk would provide only one tenth as much zinc, less than the *in utero* accumulation rate. This falling zinc concentration almost certainly plays an important part in the aetiology of the zinc deficiency seen in preterm infants (vide infra). Milk from mothers of preterm infants (Table 11.2) contains the same or slightly more zinc when compared to the milk of mothers of full term infants (13).

It has been observed that acrodermatitis enteropathica often appears at weaning when cow's milk is introduced, and may be ameliorated by giving breast milk (3). Lönnerdal *et al.* (1980) (16) have shown that, whereas most of the zinc in cow's milk is bound to casein, in human milk a higher proportion is present as zinc citrate. They suggest that this difference may result in a greater availability of zinc from breast milk.

Table 11.1. Changes in concentration of zinc in human milk during lactation.

Postpartum		μg/100 ml	$\pm$s.d.	References
1	day	825	$\pm$17	(11)
5	days	507	$\pm$14	(11)
15	days	324	$\pm$29	(11)
2–4	weeks	340	$\pm$10	(12)
2	months	210	$\pm$10	(12)
3	months	170	$\pm$10	(12)
4–7	months	80	$\pm$10	(12)

Table 11.2. Comparison of changes of zinc concentration in milk from mothers of full term and preterm infants (13).

Postpartum		Full term μg/100 ml	$\pm$s.d.	Preterm μg/100 ml	$\pm$s.d.
3–5	days	535	$\pm$120	530	$\pm$145
8–10	days	410	$\pm$65	475	$\pm$156
12–17	days	337	$\pm$60	431	$\pm$135
28–30	days	260	$\pm$65	392	$\pm$110

Formulas

The concentration of zinc in formulas from different countries is given in Table 11.3. The concentration is very variable and a few of the samples examined had levels much lower than breast milk. It would be very imprudent to feed milks with such low zinc concentrations to preterm infants. The sample(s) with a high concentration are also outside the range found in breast milk and their use would need definite justification.

Table 11.3. Zinc concentration of different infant formulas

Country of origin	No of samples	Zinc Mean	μg/100 ml Range	Reference
USA	14	428	21–1348	(14)
Sweden	12	82	9–466	(14)
West Germany	12	187	18–620	(14)
Japan	8	110	89–128	(14)
The Netherlands	2	82	44–121	(14)
England	2	192	135–249	(14)
Full term formula	9	340	210–460	(15)
Preterm formula	3	690	630–740	(15)
Soy formula	1	400		(15)
France	2	184	103–265	(14)
Norway	1	202		(14)

Zinc absorption by infants

Cavell & Widdowson (1964) (17) showed that breast-fed full term infants aged 5–8 days were in negative zinc balance averaging -230 μg/kg per day. How long such negative balances persist is now known. Dauncey *et al.* (1977) (18) studied preterm infants fed pooled pasteurized human milk with a mean zinc concentration of 336±69 μg Zn/100 ml. These infants were in negative balance on day 10 of life averaging -400 μg/kg per day (18). No infant was in positive balance before the 40th day of life and in some cases negative balance persisted until the 60th day of life. When infants such as these are discharged home it can be estimated that the total amount and concentration of zinc in their bodies is less than a normal infant of equivalent size or gestation. If they are fully breast-fed they will be receiving a diet with a falling concentration of zinc and they may become vulnerable to zinc deficiency.

Zinc deficiency in preterm infants

There are now six papers reporting nine cases of zinc deficiency occuring as a late sequel to premature birth (19,20,21,22,23,24). The infants were between 27 and 32 weeks gestation, and 975–1980 g birth weight. The onset of symptoms occurred between 2 and 4.5 months of age and the features were those given above. Most of the cases were completely breast-fed and in six the mothers' milk had a very low zinc concentration (26–58 μg/100 ml). Response to therapy was prompt with oral doses of zinc sulphate providing from 1.0 to 4.0 mg Zn/kg per day, and supplements were continued until 4.0–17.5 months of age. It is now established that preterm infants are subject to dietary zinc deficiency though it is a rare occurrence.

AVAILABLE FOODS

The changes in the concentration of zinc in breast milk have been described above (Table 11.1 and 11.2). The formulas available in the UK designed for full term infants contain 0.21–0.46 mg Zn/100 ml, whereas those intended for preterm infants contain more (0.65–0.74 mg Zn/100 ml). Two formulas in the USA, one for LBW infants and one Experimental Special Care Formula contain 0.8 and 1.22 mg Zn/100 ml respectively (25). Infants fed the latter formula had higher plasma zinc levels than those fed conventional formulas, indicating that more zinc was absorbed. However, no other benefit was demonstrated (25).

REQUIREMENTS AND ADVISABLE INTAKES

Since zinc is an essential nutrient it should be present in all milks used for infant feeding. Because the concentration in breast milk is continually declining and zinc deficiency has been observed in infants fed breast milk with a low concentration of zinc (20,23), it is not practical to imitate breast milk. Also it is not wise to design formulas with concentrations of zinc in the lower part of the range found in breast milk which are known to be associated with the occurrence of zinc deficiency. Pooled breast milk from early lactation has been shown to contain 0.36±0.07 mg Zn/100 ml (16) or 0.55 mg/100 kcal. Using this as a guide and recognizing the rarity of clinically apparent zinc deficiency in babies fed pooled human milk and current full term infant formulas when fed at 200 ml/kg per day, it is possible to state that an intake of 0.72 mg/kg per day is satisfactory for the great majority of infants. However, since dietary zinc deficiency has been reported in preterm infants it is likely that transient or subclinical deficiency may occur more frequently than at present supposed, but pass unrecognized because of difficulties in diagnosis. For these reasons a case can be made for avoiding low concentrations of zinc, and for the modest augmentation of zinc concentration (0.6–0.8 mg Zn/100 ml) found in the preterm formulas marketed in Europe which aim to provide up to 1.4 mg/kg per day. However, in the present state of knowledge this should not be mandatory.

Recommendations of other bodies

ESPGAN Committee on Nutrition: (26) (full term infants). 'minimum value 0.3 mg/100 kcal (0.2 mg/100 ml)'

Department of Health and Social Security: (27) (full term infants). 'It is therefore suggested that the concentration of zinc in a reconstituted infant feed should not be below that found in cow's milk (200 μg/100 ml) and although there is no evidence of harm from a high concentration of zinc in any formula which is at present available, the amount of zinc should not exceed the upper range of values known to occur in cow's milk (600 μg/100 ml).'

American Academy of Pediatrics: Committee on Nutrition (1976): (28) (full term infants). 'The minimum requirement for zinc. . . is approximately 0.5 mg/100 kcal (3.2 mg of zinc per litre).'

American Academy of Pediatrics: Committee on Nutrition (1977): (29) (low birth weight infants). '0.5 mg Zn. . . 100 kcals.'

Canadian Paediatric Society (1985): (30) (low birth weight infants). '. . .Studies suggest daily requirements of approximately 0.5 mg/100 kcals.'

American Academy of Pediatrics: Committee on Nutrition (1985): (31) (low birth weight infants). 'The AAP Committee on Nutrition has proposed that infant formulas for full term infants supply 0.5 mg per 100 kcal. There is no reason, at the present time to modify these recommended levels for LBW infants.'

GUIDELINES

1. With the knowledge presently available no case can be made for routinely giving supplements of zinc to breast-fed infants. It should, however, be recognized that a late deficiency, though rare, may occur in some infants.
2. A formula designed for preterm infants should contain not less than 0.55 mg Zn/100 kcal (i.e. 0.72 mg/kg per day at 130 kcal/kg per day). An upper limit cannot be recommended with any certainty but at present there seems no

reason to exceed 1.1 mg/100 kcal (i.e. 1.4 mg/kg per day at 130 kcal/kg per day). Intakes higher than this may prevent an occasional case of zinc deficiency but this has not been shown. The advantages or dangers of higher intakes have not been adequately investigated.

REFERENCES

1. Todd W.R., Elvehjem C.A. & Hart E.B. (1934). Zinc in the nutrition of the rat. *Am. J. Physiol.* **107**, 146–56.
2. Shaw J.C.L. (1979). Trace elements in the fetus and young infant. I Zinc. *Am. J. Dis. Child.* **133**, 1260–8.
3. Moynahan E.J. & Barnes P.M. (1973). Zinc deficiency and a synthetic diet for lactose intolerance. *Lancet* i, 676–7.
4. Moynahan E.H. (1974). Acrodermatitis enteropathica: a lethal inherited human zinc deficiency disorder. *Lancet* ii, 399–400.
5. Hurley L.S. (1969). Zinc deficiency in the developing rat. *Am. J. Clin. Nutr.* **22**, 1332–9.
6. Hambridge K.M., Neldner K.H. & Walravens P.A. (1975). Zinc, acrodermatitis enteropathica, and congenital malformations. *Lancet* ii, 577–8.
7. Jameson S. (1976). Effects of zinc deficiency in human reproduction. *Acta Med. Scand.* (Suppl.) **593**, 5–89.
8. Widdowson E.M. & Dickerson J.W.T. (1961). Chemical composition of the body. In: *Mineral Metabolism* (eds C.L. Comar & F. Bronner) Chapter 17. Academic Press, New York.
9. Widdowson E.M., Chan H., Harrison G.E. & Milner R.D.G. (1972). Accumulation of Cu, Zn, Mn, Cr, and Co in the human liver before birth. *Biol. Neonat.* **20**, 360–7.
10. Buhler R.H.O. & Kagi J.H.R. (1974). Human hepatic metallothioneins. *FEBS Lett.* **39**, 229–34.
11. Nassi L., Poggini G., Vicchi C. & Galvan P. (1974). Zinc, copper and iron in human colostrum and milk. *Minerva Pediatrica* **26**, 832–6.
12. Hambidge M.K. (1976). Importance of trace elements in human nutrition. *Curr. Med. Res. & Opin.* **14**, 44.
13. Mendelson R.A., Anderson G.H. & Bryan M.H. (1982). Zinc, copper and iron content of milk from mothers of preterm infants. *Early Hum. Dev.* **6**, 145–51.
14. Lönnerdal B., Stanislowski A.G. & Hurley L.S. (1980). Isolation of a low molecular weight zinc binding ligand from human milk. *J. Inorg. Biochem.* **112**, 71–8.
15. Lonnerdal B., Keen C.L., Ohtake M. & Tamura T. (1983). Iron, zinc, copper, and maganese in infant formulas. *Am. J. Dis. Child.* **137**, 433–7.
16. Shaw J.C.L. Unpublished data.
17. Cavell P.A. & Widdowson E.M. (1964). Intakes and excretions of iron, copper and zinc in the neonatal period. *Arch. Dis. Child.* **39**, 496–501.
18. Dauncey M.J., Shaw J.C.L. & Urman J. (1977). The absorption and retention of magnesium, zinc and copper by low birthweight infants fed pasteurised human breast milk. *Pediatr. Res.* **11**, 991–7.
19. Sivasubramanian K.N. & Henkin R.I. (1978). Behavioural and dermatologic changes and low serum zinc and copper concentration in two premature infants after parental alimentation. *J. Pediatr.* **93**, 847–51.
20. Aggett P.J., Atherton D.J., More J., Davey J., Delves H.T. & Harris J.T. (1980). Symptomatic zinc deficiency in a breast fed preterm infant. *Arch. Dis. Child.* **55**, 547–50.
21. Bonifazi E., Rigillo N., DeSimone B. & Meneghini C.L. (1980). Acquired dermatitis due to zinc deficiency in a premature infant. *Act. Der. Ven.* **60**, 449–51.

22. Blom I., Jameson S., Kroom F., Larsson-Styme B. & Wranne L. (1981). Zinc deficiency in a boy of low birth weight. *Br. J. Dermatol.* **104**, 459–64.
23. Zimmerman A.W., Hambridge K.M., Lepow M., Greenberg R.D., Storer M.L. & Casey C.E. (1982). Acrodermatitis in breast fed premature infants: Evidence for a defect or mammary zinc secretion. *Pediatrics* **69**, 176–83.
24. Weymouth R.D. & Czarneki D. (1981). Symptomatic zinc deficiency in premature breast fed infants associated with defective mammary gland zinc secretion. *Austr. Paediatr. J.* **17**, 131.
25. Proc 2nd Ross Clin Res Conf. (1982). *Meeting Nutritional Goals for Low Birth Weight Infants.* Ross Laboratories, Columbus, Ohio.
26. ESPGAN Committee on Nutrition: Guidelines on Infant Nutrition (1977). I. Recommendation for the Composition of an Adapted Formula. *Acta. Paediatr. Scand.* (Suppl.) **262**.
27. Department of Health and Social Security (1980). Report on Health and Social Subjects. No. 18. Artificial feeds for the young infant. HMSO, London.
28. American Academy of Pediatrics: Committee in Nutrition (1976). Commentary on breast feeding and infant formulas, including proposed standards for formulas. *Pediatrics* **57**, 278–85.
29. American Academy of Pediatrics: Committee on Nutrition (1977). Nutritional needs of low birth weight infants. *Pediatrics* **60**, 519–30.
30. Canadian Paediatric Society: Committee on Nutrition (1981). Feeding the low birth weight infant. *Can. Med. Ass.* **124**, 1301–11.
31. American Academy of Pediatrics: Committee on Nutrition (1985). Nutritional needs of low birthweight infants. *Pediatrics* **75**, 976–86.

12

Copper

NUTRITIONAL BACKGROUND

In 1928 Hart *et al.* (1) demonstrated that copper was essential for erythropoiesis in the rat. It is now known that copper is a component of several enzymes. These enzymes bind between 1 and 6 gram atoms of copper per mole and are mostly associated with electron transfer. Copper is essential to their activity (2,3).

Copper deficiency

The characteristics of copper deficiency in infants have been well described by Ashkenazi *et al.* (1973) (4). Many of the features can be explained on the basis of deficiency of particular copper enzymes. The prominent scalp veins and bone changes are thought to be due to impaired collagen cross linking due to depressed lysyl oxidase activity. The hypopigmentation is probably due to depressed tyrosinase activity and impaired melanin synthesis. The sideroblastic anaemia is less well understood, but there seems to be depression of iron transport into the mitochondria, and impaired incorporation of iron into protoporphyrin IX within the mitochondria. The cause of the neutropoenia is not understood.

Copper in the fetal body

The concentration of copper in the body of the fetus increases from about 3.5 mg/kg fat free body tissue at about 20 weeks gestation to about 4.8 mg/kg fat free tissue at term (5). Copper accumulates in the fetus at a rate of 51.0 μg/kg per day (6) and full term infants contain 14.4 ± 0.4 mg of copper (5). About half of this is present in the liver at a mean concentration of 6.4 mg/100 g wet weight (7) where it is bound to metallothionein (8). Some of the metallothionein bound copper is excreted in the bile following birth but the remainder probably forms a reserve. Since preterm infants contain less copper than full term infants, the concentration of copper in their bodies will fall unless they receive and absorb sufficient copper from their milk.

150

Copper absorption by infants

Cavell & Widdowson (1964) (9) studied 10 full term infants given breast milk containing 62 ± 0.8 μg/100 ml of copper. Seven of the infants were in negative balance which averaged for the whole group -9 μg/kg per day (range -66 to $+29$ μg/kg per day). How long these negative balances persist is not known but it is interesting that they occurred at a time when the milk copper concentration was at its highest. Dauncey *et al.* (1977) (10) have shown that preterm infants fed pooled human breast milk with a mean copper content of 41 μg/100 ml were in negative balance of -36 μg/kg per day between day 10 and 12 of life, and two infants fed SMA were in a negative balance on day ten of -58 and -50 μg/kg per day respectively (Shaw J.C.L. Unpublished data). Of the six infants given breast milk all but one were in positive copper balance by the 40th day of life.

Copper deficiency in preterm infants

The conditions outlined above — namely, low total body copper, malabsorption, and a low concentration in milk together with rapid growth — all contribute to the development of copper defiiciency in preterm infants. There are now five papers reporting six cases of copper deficiency in preterm infants (4,11,12,13,14) and others where the diagnosis was suspected but not established (15,16). It is probably significant that all the infants were given a variety of formulas and none of them were breast fed. The concentrations of caeruloplasmin and of copper in the blood did not correspond as they should, in some of the reports, and this probably reflects the difficulty of analysing plasma copper. It seems likely, however, that the severe features become evident when the plasma copper falls below 20 μg/100 ml and the caeruloplasmin levels are below 5 μg/100 ml. Response to treatment was prompt with doses of copper between 0.6 and 0.8 mg/kg per day given as 1% solution of copper sulphate.

It should be emphasized that the plasma copper and caeruloplasmin are normally low in preterm infants at birth and though they increase with post-conceptional age low values will be encountered at 47–48 weeks of post-conceptional age in some infants (17). There is no evidence that such low levels taken alone are evidence of copper deficiency.

AVAILABLE FOODS

Breast milk

The changes in the concentration of copper in human milk during lactation are given in the Tables 12.1 and 12.2. According to these data (18,19,20) the concentration changes little during lactation although Vuori & Kuitunen (1979) (21) have shown a threefold fall in mean milk copper level from 60 μg/100 ml during the second week of lactation to about 25 μg/100 ml after six months. Some of their late milk samples had a very low copper level and might well contain insufficient copper for an infant born prematurely. The milk from mothers of preterm infants (Table 12.2) had the same or slightly higher concentrations of copper compared with the milk of mothers of full term infants (20). Therefore milk from an infant's own mother containing 74 μg/100 ml (20) would provide about 148 μg/kg per day if given at 200 ml/kg per day during the first month of life but the intake would decline to about 120 μg/kg per day at three months of life (19).

Table 12.1 Changes in concentration of copper in human milk during lactation

Postpartum	μg/100 ml ±s.d.		
2– 5 days	46	±18	(18)
6–13 days	67	±19	(18)
15–28 days	58	± 8	(18)
2 months	61	±16	(19)
3 months	42	±22	(19)
4– 7 months	29	±23	(19)

Table 12.2 Comparison of changes in copper concentration in milk from mothers of full term and preterm infants (20).

Postpartum	Full term μg/100 ml ±s.d.		Preterm μg/100 ml ±s.d.	
3– 5 days	72	±13	83	±21
8–10 days	73	±21	78	±18
12–17 days	57	± 8	75	±24
28–30 days	58	± 9	63	±14

Formulas

The concentration of copper in different infant formulas is given in Table 12.3. The concentration is very variable, it rarely exceeds the amount present in breast milk and some milks had almost undetectable amounts of copper. The formulas for full term infants available in the UK with added copper had concentrations ranging from 47 to 63 μg/100 ml, while those without added copper had concentrations ranging from 1.0 to 3.8 μg/100 ml. These milks had not been fortified with copper because they were not packed under nitrogen, and the addition of copper would have lead to oxidative changes. It cannot be recommended that milks with such low copper levels should ever be fed to preterm infants but if they are, their low copper content should be recognized and the infants checked for signs of copper deficiency. Some formulas designed for preterm infants contain higher levels of copper, in the range 60–80 μg/100 ml. In the USA even higher levels may be found. For example, in an experimental low birth weight special care formula the concentration is 202 μg/100 ml. However, studies with a formula augmented to a copper concentration of 167 μg/100 ml did not result in any increase in the plasma copper or caeruloplasmin levels during 3 months when compared to a control formula with 40 μg Cu/100 ml (24).

Table 12.3. Copper concentration of different infant formulas

Country of origin	No of samples	Copper Mean	μg/100 ml Range	Reference
USA	14	48	31–65	(22)
Sweden	12	18	3–70	(22)
West Germany	12	20	1–135	(22)
Japan	8	6	2–15	(22)
The Netherlands	2	28	14–43	(22)
England	2	14	5–23	(22)
Full term formula	9	18	1–47	(23)
Preterm formula	3	68	62–73	(23)
Soy formula	1	51		(23)
France	2	12	5–20	(22)
Norway	1	25		(22)

REQUIREMENTS AND ADVISABLE INTAKES

Copper is an essential nutrient and should be present in all milks used for infant feeding. Copper deficiency is known to occur as a sequel to premature birth in infants fed formulas, therefore low levels of copper in formula milks should be avoided. In spite of the negative copper balance following birth copper deficiency has not been reported in infants fed breast milk, so it would seem reasonable to supplement formulas to give a concentration of copper within the upper part of the range (from the mean to +s.d) of that found in breast milk in the late part of the neonatal period (i.e. 90–120 μg/100 kcal).

Recommendations of other bodies

ESPGAN Committee on Nutrition (1977): (25) (full term infants). Minimum value 30 μg/100 kcal (20 μg/100 ml).

Department of Health and Social Security (1980): (26) (full term infants). 'It seems likely that the amount of copper in infant feeds should be not more and not less than the amounts present on average in mature human and cow's milk, that is to say not less than 10 μg and not more than 60 μg/100 ml, but at present sufficient information is not available for a recommendation to be made.'

American Academy of Pediatrics (1976): (27). Minimum intake 90 μg/100 kcal.

American Academy of Pediatrics (1977): (28). 'Recent data suggests that an intake of 90 μg/100 kcal is desirable.'

Canadian Paediatric Society (1981): (29). 'It has been suggested that low birth weight infants require 90 μg/100 kcal to avoid copper depletion.'

American Academy of Pediatrics (1985): (30). '90 μg/100 kcal continues to be appropriate.'

GUIDELINES

1.   At present there seems to be no case for routinely supplementing breast-fed infants with copper.
2.   Formulas designed for preterm infants should provide at least 90 μg/100 kcal (i.e. 117 μg/kg per day at 130 kcal/kg per day). An upper limit cannot be recommended with certainty but there seems no reason to exceed the amounts present in mature human milk, that is about 120 μg/100 kcal.
3.   This recommendation should be subject to re-evaluation when more data become available. Higher intakes may prevent some cases of deficiency but this has not been established, and the possible dangers of higher intakes have not been fully examined.

REFERENCES

1. Hart E.B., Steenbock H., Waddell J. & Elvehjem C.A. (1982). Iron in nutrition. VII Copper as a supplement to iron for haemoglobin building in the rat. *J. Biol. Chem.* 77, 797–812.
2. O'Dell B. (1976). Biochemistry and physiology of copper in vertebrates. In: *Trace Elements in Human Health and Disease.* Vol 1. (eds A.S. Prasad & D. Oberleas) pp. 391–413. Academic Press, New York.
3. Lee G.E., Williams D.M. & Cartwright G.E. (1976). Role of copper in iron metabolism and heme biosynthesis. In: *Trace Elements in Human Health and Disease.* Vol 1. (eds A.S. Prasad & D. Oberleas) pp. 373–90. Academic Press, New York.
4. Asheknzai A., Levine S., Dialjetti M., Fishel E. & Benvenisti O. (1973). The syndrome of neonatal copper deficiency. *Pediatrics* 52, 525–33.

5. Widdowson E.M. & Dickerson J.W.T. (1961). Chemical composition of the body. In: *Mineral Metabolism* Vol. 2 (eds C.L. Comar & F. Bruhner) Chapter 17. Academic Press, New York.
6. Shaw J.C.L. (1980). Trace elements in the fetus and young infant. II. Copper, Manganese, Selenium and Chromium. *Am. J. Dis. Child.* **134**, 74–81.
7. Widdowson E.M., Chan H., Harrison G.E. & Milner R.D.G. (1972). Accumulation of Cu, Zn, Mn, Cr, and Co in the human liver before birth. *Biol. Neonat.* **20**, 360–7.
8. Ryden L. & Deutsch H.F. (1978). Preparation and properties of the major copper binding component in human fetal liver. Its identification as metallothionein. *J. Biol. Chem.* **253**, 519–24.
9. Cavell P.A. & Widdowson E.M. (1964). Intakes and excretions of iron, Copper and zinc in the neonatal period. *Arch. Dis. Child.* **39**, 496–501.
10. Dauncey M.J., Shaw J.C.L. & Urman J. (1977). The absorption and retention of magnesium, zinc and copper by low birth weight infants fed pasteurised human breast milk. *Pediatr. Res.* **11**, 991–7.
11. Al-Rashid R.A. & Spangler J. (1971). Neonatal copper deficiency. *N. Eng. J. Med.* **285**, 841–3.
12. Seely J.R., Humphrey G.B. & Matler B.J. (1972). Copper deficiency in a premature infant fed on iron fortified formula. *N. Eng. J. Med.* **286**, 109.
13. Yuen P., Liu H.J. & Hutchinson J.H. (1979). Copper deficiency in a low birth weight infant. *Arch. Dis. Child.* **54**, 553–4.
14. Blumenthal I., Lealman G.T. & Franklyn P.P. (1980). Fracture of the femur, fish odour, and copper deficiency in a preterm infant. *Arch. Dis. Child.* **55**, 229–31.
15. Heller R.M., Kirchner S.G., O'Neill J.A. Jr., Hough A.J. Jr., Howard K.M. Kramer S.S. & Green H.L. (1978). Skeletal changes of copper deficiency in infants receiving prolonged total parenteral nutrition. *J. Pediatr.* **92**, 947–9.
16. Sturgeon P. & Brubacker C. (1956). Copper deficiency in infants. A syndrome characterised by hypocupraemia iron deficiency and hyproteinaemia. *Am. J. Dis. Child.* **92**, 254–65.
17. Hillman L.S. (1981). Serial serum copper concentrations in premature and SGA infants during the first three months of life. *J. Pediatr.* **98**, 305–8.
18. Stolley H., Galgan V. & Droese W. (1981). Nahr- und Wirkstoffe in Frauenmilch: Protein, Laktose, Mineralen, Spurenelementi und Thiamin. *Monatsschr. Kinderheilkd.* **129**, 293–7.
19. Hambidge M.K. (1976). Importance of trace elements in human nutrition. *Curr. Med. Res. & Opin.* **4**, 44.
20. Mendelson R.A., Anderson G.H. & Bryan M.H. (1982). Zinc, copper and iron content of milk from mothers of preterm infants. *Early Hum. Dev.* **6**, 145–51.
21. Vuori F. & Kuitunen P. (1979). The concentration of copper and zinc in human milk. *Acta Paediatr. Scand.* **68**, 33–7.
22. Lönnerdal B., Keen C.L., Ohtake M. & Tamura T. (1983). Iron, zinc, copper, and manganese in infant formulas. *Am. J. Dis. Child.* **137**, 433–7.
23. Shaw J.C.L. Unpublished data.
24. Hillman L.S., Martin L. & Fiore B. (1981). Effect of oral copper supplementation on serum copper and ceruloplasmin concentrations in premature infants. *J. Pediatr.* **98**, 311–3.
25. ESPGAN Committee on Nutrition: Guidelines on Infant Nutrition (1977). I. Recommendation for the Composition of an Adapted Formula. *Acta Paediatr. Scand.* (Suppl.) **262**.
26. Department of Health and Social Security (1980). Report on Health and Social Subjects. No. 18. Artificial Feeds for the Young Infant. HMSO, London.
27. American Academy of Pediatrics: Committee in Nutrition (1976). Commentary on breast feeding and infant formulas, including proposed standards for formulas. *Pediatrics* **57**, 278–85.
28. American Academy of Pediatrics: Committee on Nutrition (1977). Nutritional Needs of Low Birth Weight Infants. *Pediatrics* **60**, 519–30.
29. Canadian Paediatric Society: Committee on Nutrition (1981). Feeding the Low Birth Weight

Infant. *Can. Med. Ass.* **124**, 1301–11.
30. American Academy of Pediatrics: Committee on Nutrition (1985). Nutritional needs of low birth weight infants. *Pediatrics* 75, 976–86.

13
Other Trace Elements

MANGANESE

Nutritional background

Manganese is an essential nutrient for mammals and is a component of pyruvate carboxylase and mitochondrial superoxide dismutase. Manganese is also an activator of hydrolases, kinases, decarboxylases, and transferases. The metabolism of manganese has been reviewed by Leach (1976) (1). The total amount of manganese in the human fetus is unknown so the intrauterine accumulation rate cannot be estimated. However, the concentration ranges from $0.67 \pm 0.16 \, \mu g/g$ dry weight in skeletal muscle to $4.3 \pm 1.6 \, \mu g/g$ dry weight in the liver (2,3). The concentration does not change with gestational age.

Manganese deficiency

Manganese deficiency has been described in numerous species and the principal manifestations are impaired growth, skeletal abnormalities, depressed reproductive function and, in the newborn, ataxia. Morphological changes occur in the mitochondria associated with reduced oxygen consumption and abnormalities are also apparent in the endoplasmic reticulum. There is evidence that the skeletal abnormalities, and the abnormalities in the otolith organ responsible for the ataxia in the newborn (4), are both the result of disorded chondrogenesis. This is thought to be due to impairment of the activity of glycosyl transferases involved in mucopolysaccharide synthesis.

There has been no well documented case of manganese deficiency in man. In one adult case report where manganese deficiency was suspected the subject developed a mild dermatitis, slight reddening of the beard, and depression of vitamin K dependent clotting factors resistant to treatment with vitamin K (5).

Manganese in milk

Breast milk

The amounts of manganese reported by different authors to be present in breast milk are variable (6). McLeod & Robinson (1972) (6) from New Zealand report an average value of 1.5 (range 1.2–2.0)μg/100 ml. Vuori & Kuitunen (1979) (7) from Finland found an average value of 0.78 (range 0.18–1.78)μg/100 ml, and in milk from the second week of lactation the median value was 0.59 μg/100 ml and 50% of the values fell between 0.49–0.7 μg/100 ml. The median fell to 0.4 μg/100 ml by the second month of lactation and then remained constant (7). Vaughan *et al.* (1979) (8) from the USA studied milk from the 1st to the 31st month of lactation and found values that ranged from 1.41±0.51 to 2.53±0.39 μg/100 ml and they found no decline with lactation.

Cow's milk and infant formulas

The manganese content of cow's milk is higher than that of breast milk and has been reported to be 4.0 (range 3.2–5.4)μg/100 ml (7). The amounts present in infant formulas are much more variable. Mean values for formulas obtained from different countries are given in Table 13.1. Some of the means are probably unrepresentatively high because of the skew distribution of results. It is noteworthy that some of the formulas contain 100–1000 times as much manganese as human milk.

Table 13.1. Manganese concentration of different infant formulas.

Country of origin	No of samples	Manganese Mean	μg/100 ml Range	Reference
USA	14	108	20–780	(9)
Sweden	12	57	0–190	(9)
West Germany	12	57	0–368	(9)
Japan	8	6	4–13	(9)
The Netherlands	2	8	3–14	(9)
England	2	3	1–5	(9)
Full term formula	12	7	3–18	(10)
Preterm formula	3	20	6–35	(10)
Soy formula	1	131		(10)
France	2	4	3–5	(9)
Norway	1	10		(9)

Manganese absorption by newborn babies

Widdowson (1969) (11) reported that breast-fed full term infants aged 5–8 days excreted five times as much manganese in their stools as they received in their milk and were therefore in negative balance. The source of the endogenous manganese was almost certainly the bile (1). The inability of the newborn infants to reabsorb the manganese may be due to lack of enzymes necessary to liberate manganese from complexes present in the bile (11).

Nothing is known about manganese absorption by preterm infants but it is quite possible that they would be in negative manganese balance for some time after birth. The concentration of manganese in the hair of both full term and preterm infants declines with postnatal age but at 12 months of age it is significantly lower in the preterm infants compared with the full term infants (12). This may indicate that preterm infants have less manganese in their bodies due perhaps to malabsorption following birth.

Requirements and advisable intakes

Since no case of manganese deficiency has been reported in infants it must be assumed that the amounts present in human milk and most infant formulas are satisfactory. However, the effects of the very high concentrations such as those found in some soy formulas are now known and such formulas should be used with caution in preterm infants.

Recommendations of other bodies

ESPGAN Committee on Nutrition: (13) (full term infants). 'The values recommended below are those given by Codex Alimentarius'
'Manganese
Minimum value 5 μg/100 kcal (3.4 μg/100 ml)
Maximum value non specified.'

Department of Health and Social Security: (14) (full term infants). '. . . the manganese content of artificial feeds should be within the range of that found in human milk and in infant formulas which are now available.'

American Academy of Pediatrics: (15) 'The committee recommends 5 μg/100 kcal of formula, approximately the level in commonly used milk based infant formulas.'

American Academy of Pediatrics: (16). 'The Committee on Nutrition has recently proposed that infant formulas for full term infants supply. . . 5 μg manganese per 100 kcal. There is no basis for modifying levels for low birth weight infants.'

Canadian Paediatric Society: (17) 'The recommended requirement for manganese for infant formulas is 5 μg/100 kcal, one study of parenteral nutrition suggested that this may be low and 10 μg/100 kcal was recommended.'

American Academy of Pediatrics: Committee on Nutrition (1985) (18) (low birth weight infants). 'The Committee on Nutrition has recently proposed that infant formulas for full term infants supply. . . 5 μg manganese per 100 kcal. There is no basis for modifying levels for low birth weight infants.'

Guidelines

Manganese is an essential nutrient and should be present in all milks used for infant feeding. The concentration of manganese in a formula designed for preterm infants should not be lower than the average value found in human milk, that is about 1.5 μg/100 ml (2.1 μg/100 kcal). An upper limit cannot be set in the present state of knowledge. Though there are many formulas that have been safely used that contain more manganese than human milk there seems no reason to exceed the amounts found in cow's milk namely 5.4 μg/100 ml (7.5 μg/100 kcal). Some formulas contain very high concentrations of manganese, >100 times that found in breast milk. Although this is not known to be harmful we do not recommend giving such milks to LBW infants.

SELENIUM

Nutritional background

Selenium (Se) is a component of glutathione peroxidase (GSH-Px) (19,20). It catalyses the reduction of hydrogen peroxide using glutathione as a proton donor and serves to protect the cell membrane against peroxide induced damage. In animals both GSH-Px and vitamin E share similar functions, as both substances act directly or indirectly as natural antioxidants that protect cell membranes against lipid peroxidation (21). However, it is not known to what extent vitamin E can compensate for a deficiency of Se or vice versa.

The Se concentration in the liver of preterm infants at birth (1.21±0.17 μg/g dry wt.) is higher than that of full term infants (0.93±0.16 μg/g dry wt.) whereas in the heart it is about the same. After birth the concentration decreases (22).

Table 13.2. Selenium content of tissues of full term infants (122).

Tissue	At birth	Aged 1–9 months	Aged 1–6 years
Liver (μg/g dry wt.)	0.93±0.16	0.58±0.21	0.59±0.10
Heart (μg/g dry wt.)	0.67±0.33	0.46±0.36	0.29±0.01

The published values for the Se content of erythrocytes and the activity of glutathione peroxidase in newborn infants are contradictory. Several workers have shown that GSH-Px activities are lower in erythrocytes of newborn full term and LBW infants than in the erythrocytes of adults (19) though peroxide induced haemolysis was comparable to that of adults (23). However, this could not be confirmed by Lombeck *et al.* (25) who found similar activity in cord blood and adult's erythrocytes. Hågå & Lunde (24) found approximately the same Se content in erythrocytes of newborn full term, LBW, and small for gestational age infants.

The serum selenium concentration is higher in full term infants fed human milk than in infants fed adapted formulas (26,27) and this is presumably due to the higher levels found in human milk (see below). In LBW infants the serum Se concentration at birth is lower than in full term infants (24,28). It decreases further during the months following birth, as do the erythrocyte GSH-Px and the Se content of hair (25,29). This decline may be due to the falling Se concentration of human milk and the lower concentration in cow's milk (30,31). In spite of the falling serum concentrations, however, clinical symptoms of Se deficiency have never been found in LBW infants either at birth or later on.

Deficiency

The symptoms of Keshan disease seem to be the clinical signs of severe selenium deficiency (32). This is a cardiomyopathy with a high mortality which affects mainly children and pregnant women and it occurs in localized areas of China where the soil and hence the staple diet (principally cereals) is deficient in Se. The mortality and incidence of the disease have been reduced to zero by distributing large scale supplements of sodium selenite, 0.5–1.0 mg/day. Some areas of Europe have low soil selenium concentrations, and though selenium deficiency has not been reported from Europe it may yet be identified. There have also been three reports of similar symptomatology in patients on long term total parenteral nutrition (33,34,35). However, patients with phenylketonuria treated with artificial diets with low selenium content develop reduced concentrations of selenium in their plasma, erythrocytes and hair, and a marked reduction in glutathione peroxidase activity in plasma and erythrocytes, without any clinical signs of deficiency (36,37). It is therefore possible that there is an additional factor, deficient in Keshan disease which enhances the effect of the selenium deficiency, for example vitamin E deficiency.

In toddlers with low GSH-Px activity in serum and erythrocytes normal levels are restored by giving 2.4–2.9 ng Se/kcal in the form of selenium enriched yeast (37).

Selenium in milk

All reports agree that the concentration of selenium declines throughout lactation. There are, however, big regional variations in the concentrations of selenium in human milk. Table 13.3 gives the levels found in human milk in Japan.

Table 13.3. Changes in concentration of selenium in human milk in Japan (31).

Stage of lactation	ng/ml	Range
Colostrum	80	35–152
1 week	29	15–79
1 month	18	9–39
5 months	18	9–33

Similar concentrations have been found in the USA (30) and rather higher concentrations have been found in mature milk in Central Europe which range from 13.9 to 59.4 ng Se/ml (30). In Belgium, however, much lower values have been reported (38) and are shown in Table 13.4.

Table 13.4. Changes in concentration of selenium in human milk in Belgium (38).

Stage of lactation	Selenium ng/g Median	Range
0–3 days	15	6.6–27.2
5–7 days	11	5.5–18.7
8–10 days	13	6.7–17.7
30 days	9	6.7–12.7
60 days	9	5.6–15.4

Pooled human milk (mean ± s.d.) 9.3 ± 1.3

These values are rather similar to those reported for breast milk of Finnish women, which declined from 10.7 ng Se/ml at one month to 5.6 ng Se/ml at six months of lactation (39). The values for liquid cow's milk and infant formulas range from 6.7 to 13.8 ng Se/ml (27,30).

Requirements and advisable intakes

Because signs of clinical Se deficiency have not been found in LBW infants the Se intake from human milk or cow's milk and infant formulas seems to be adequate for growth. The postnatal decrease, in the selenium content of hair (29) and blood (25), and in the GSH-Px activity of erythrocytes (25) are unexplained. It does not necessarily imply deficiency, or provide grounds for supplementing the diet. The addition of selenium to food is not without problems because most selenium compounds are toxic if given in excess.

Recommendations of other bodies

ESPGAN Committee on Nutrition: (40) (full term infants). No recommendation.

Department of Health and Social Security: (41) (full term infants). 'The amounts (of selenium) in human milk and in infant feeds which are in use at present are presumably adequate. . . and no recommendations are made.'

American Academy of Pediatrics: (42). No recommendation.

American Academy of Pediatrics: (43). '. . . no information on which to base recommendations at this time.'

Canadian Paediatric Society: (44). 'Presumably standard formulas and human milk provide adequate quantities.'

American Academy of Pediatrics (1985): (45). No recommendation.

Guidelines

Selenium is an essential nutrient and should be present in formulas designed for preterm infants. However, in the present state of knowledge, it is not possible to give any guidelines and in view of the possible toxicity of selecium salts we do not recommend that selenium supplements be given at the present time.

MOLYBDENUM

Nutritional background

Molybdenum is a component of a cofactor essential for the function of xanthine dehydrogenase, sulphite oxidase, aldehyde oxidase, and nitrate reductase (46,47). Molybdenum cofactors common to these enzymes have been isolated from a variety of plant and animal sources. Since they have similar properties, and seem functionally interchangeable, they are thought to be identical (48). From this it can be inferred that molybdenum is an essential element for man.

Deficiency

An infant who has been shown to be missing the molybdenum cofactor (49,50) presented with mental retardation, cerebral atrophy, dislocated ocular lenses, nystagmus and fits. Examination of the patient's blood showed elevated levels of xanthine with low levels of uric acid. There were elevated levels of sulphite, thiosulphite, S-sulphocysteine and taurine in the urine with reduced amounts of sulphate. Similar biochemical findings have been reported in an adult patient on total parenteral nutrition who responded to molybdate supplementation (51). These features are entirely consistent with known functions of the enzymes requiring the molybdenum cofactor. Deficiency has not been reported in the premature infant.

Molybdenum in milk

The only reference to the molybdenum content of human milk in the literature gives a range of 10–50 p.p.m. in milk ash. Assuming an average milk ash of 2.0 g/l this would be equivalent to about 2–10 μg/100 ml in whole milk (52). Cow's milk has been reported to contain 3.9±0.96 μg/100 ml (53) and 2.9±3.4 μg/100 ml (54). However, the molybdenum content of cow's milk depends very much on the molybdenum content of the pasture or feed they are fed on. Mean values for cow's milk range from 2.9 to 7.3 μg/100 ml and values as low as 1.8 μg/100 ml and as high as 14.7 μg/100 ml have been reported (55). No values for molybdenum in infant formulas are available.

Requirements and advisable intakes

Since molybdenum deficiency has not been described in preterm infants, and the concentration of molybdenum in infant formulas are not known it is not possible to make firm recommendations. However, molybdenum is an essential element which is present in human milk and it should be present in infant formulas.

Guidelines

It is impossible to formulate guidelines in the present state of knowledge but the committee do think that molybdenum free formulas should be avoided and that the amounts present in human milk should be used as a guide.

CHROMIUM

Nutritional background

Chromium is the most recent addition to the trace elements shown to be essential to man. However, the investigation of chromium metabolism has proved to be no simple matter and the interested reader should consult the books and reviews in the references (55–58). In particular, the chemical analysis of chromium in biological materials is very difficult and the values reported in recent years by those concerned with improving analytical methods are so much lower than those published previously that many of the earlier values are thought to be wrong (58). Chromium is present in all tissues of the body but is found in particularly high concentration in nucleic acids and in certain regions of the brain such as the caudate nucleus. From its chemical properties it has been suggested that chromium may act by stabilizing the tertiary structure of nucleoproteins, or by binding enzymes to their active sites (55).

Chromium in the fetus

Little is known about chromium in fetal development. In the rat $^{51}Cr^{3+}$ is said to cross the placenta poorly but an organic chromium complex, known as Glucose Tolerance Factor or GTF labelled with ^{51}Cr is reported to cross rapidly into the fetus (55) (but see below). Recently it has been shown that $^{51}Cr^{3+}$ given intravenously to pregnant rats is taken up by the fetoplacental unit (59). In man placental transfer must occur because chromium is present in the liver of the fetus (60). The concentration is thought to decrease during pregnancy and after birth.

Chromium deficiency

Chromium deficiency in animals is characterized by impaired glucose tolerance with fasting hyperglycaemia, glycosuria, hypercholesterolaemia, corneal opacities, impaired growth, decreased sperm count and infertility (61). These features can be reversed by giving trivalent chromium (Cr^{3+}) and also by much smaller amounts of Cr^{3+} given as an organic complex known as GTF which has been extracted from brewers yeast (55). The structure of GTF is unknown. In a partially purified form (64) containing chromium it has been shown to increase the uptake of glucose by yeast cells (63) and is thought to potentiate the action of insulin. However, Haylock *et al.* (1983) (64,65) have recently shown that many of the chromium complexes found in yeast extracts are formed in the growth medium and have no biological activity. Furthermore in the fractions found in the yeast that did have biological activity they found that the biological activity and the chromium could be separated from each other. There is some doubt therefore about the part played by GTF in the glucose intolerance of chromium deficiency.

Two cases whose symptoms were thought to be due to chromium deficiency have been described in man (66,67). Both were adult patients who had been maintained on long term parenteral nutrition providing a low chromium intake, and they both developed a severe diabetes-like illness requiring large doses of insulin. In addition one case had a peripheral neuropathy and the other a confusional state. Glucose tolerance became normal and insulin requirements fell to zero in both cases on supplementation with inorganic Cr^{3+}.

Available foods

Chromium in milk

According to Kumpulainen & Vuori (68) the concentration of chromium in breast milk falls from 0.43 ± 0.13 ng/ml between 8–18 days of lactation to 0.34 ± 0.12 ng/ml between 128–159 days of lactation. They calculated that a term infant would receive about 70 ng/kg per day of chromium. Neither the chemical form of this chromium or its bioavailability are known.

Requirements and advisable intakes

Recommendation of other bodies

No recommendations for infants have been made.

Recommendations of this committee

Chromium is thought to be an essential element for man, but deficiency has not been described in breast-fed or formula-fed infants. Because of this, and because of the analytical problems in the measurement of chromium in biological materials that still exist, it is not possible to recommend a chromium concentration for formulas designed for preterm infants.

Guidelines

In the absence of data no guidelines are possible.

IODINE

Nutritional background

Almost the entire body of iodine is concentrated in the thyroid. It is specifically required as a component of thyroglobulin and the thyroid hormones. Iodine deficiency occurs in areas where the natural iodine content of the soil is low, and in these areas iodine-deficiency cretinism is, or has been, endemic. Severe maternal iodine deficiency during pregnancy may result in the birth of infants with irreversible changes which include mental deficiency with deaf mutism and neuromuscular disorders (69), or stunted growth and hypothyroidism (70).

There is no evidence that breast or formula-fed infants ever become iodine deficient in North America, but in some parts of Europe moderate iodine deficiency may account for the syndrome of transient hypothyroidism which has been reported in premature infants (71).

Requirements and advisable intake

The iodine content of human milk is 20–120 μg/l (mean 70) (72,73) which is presumably adequate since signs of deficiency do not occur outside areas of endemic cretinism. Formulas should therefore contain no less than 40 μg/l (6 μg/100 kcal). Excess maternal iodine intake during pregnancy is associated with increased neonatal mortality (74) but there are no data on which to base an upper limit of iodine intake in the preterm infant. The iodine content of cow's milk varies considerably with the cow's diet and teat disinfection and may reach concentrations as high as 800 μg/l (75). However, in most instances the concentration is less than 300 μg/l and we would be wary of giving amounts in excess of this.

Guidelines

1 Human milk provides adequate iodine provided that the dietary intake in pregnancy and lactation is normal ($\sim$50 μg/day).
2 Formulas should not contain less than 10 μg iodine per 100 kcal (7.0 μg/dl) nor more than 45 μg/dl).

FLUORINE

Nutritional background

Fluorine is an essential trace element found mostly in bones and teeth, with traces in thyroid gland and skin. Fluoride deficiency is associated with dental caries. Fluoride excess causes fluorosis, resulting in mottling and weakening of the dental enamel, and skeletal osteosclerosis and exostoses. Fluoride apparently only crosses the placenta in minute amounts, even if the mother is taking fluoride supplements, and is present in human milk in concentrations less than 0.05 mg/litre (76) irrespective of the fluoride content of the drinking water. There is no published information about the desirable fluorine intake of preterm infants.

Requirements and advisable intake

We are unable to make any recommendations on the desirable level of fluorine intake. It can be assumed that the amount present in human milk and formula is probably sufficient to meet the minimal requirement for bone and teeth formation.

REFERENCES

1. Leach R.M. Jr. (1976). Metabolism and function of manganese. In: *Trace Elements in Human Health and Disease*, Vol. 2 (eds A.S. Prasad & D. Oberleas) pp 235–47. Academic Press, New York.
2. Casey C.E. & Robinson M.F. (1978). Copper, manganese, zinc, nickle, cadmium, and lead in human fetal tissues. *Br. J. Nutr.* 39, 639–46.
3. Widdowson E.M., Chan H., Harrison G.E. & Milner R.D.G. (1972). Accumulation of Cu, Zn, Mn, Cr & Co in human liver before birth. *Biol. Neonat.* 20, 360–7.
4. Erway L.C., Fraser A.S. & Hurley L.S. (1971). Prevention of congenital otolith defect in pallid mutant mice by manganese supplementation. *Genetics* 67, 97–108.
5. Doisy E.A. Jr. (1973). Micronutrient controls in biosynthesis of clotting proteins and cholesterol. In: *Trace Substances in Environmental Health*, Vol. 4. (ed. D.D. Hemphill) pp. 193–9. University of Missouri, Columbia.
6. Vuori E. (1979). A longitudinal study of manganese in human milk. *Acta Paediatr. Scand.* 68, 571–3.
7. McLeod B.E. & Robinson M.F. (1972). Dietary intake of manganese by New Zealand infants during the first 6 months of life. *Br. J. Nutr.* 27, 229–32.
8. Vaughan L.A., Weber C.W. & Kemberling S.R. (1979). Longitudinal changes in the mineral content of human milk. *Am. J. Clin. Nutr.* 32, 2301–6.
9. Lönnerdal B., Keen C.L., Ohtake M. & Tamura T. (1983). Iron, zinc, copper, and manganese in infant formulas. *Am. J. Dis. Child.* 137, 433–7.
10. Shaw J.C.L. Unpublished data.

11. Widdowson E.M. (1976). Trace elements in human development. In: *Mineral Metabolism in Pediatrics.* (eds D. Barltrop & W.L. Burland) pp 85–95. Blackwell Scientific Publications, Oxford.
12. Friel J.K., Gibson R.S., Balassa R. & Watts J.L. (1984). A comparison of the zinc, copper and manganese status of very low birth weight preterm and full term infants during the first 12 months. *Acta Paediatr. Scand.* **73**, 596–601.
13. ESPGAN Committee on Nutrition: Guidelines on Infant Nutrition (1977). I. Recommendation for the Composition of an Adapted Formula. *Acta Paediatr. Scand.* (Suppl.) **262**.
14. Department of Health and Social Security. Report on Health and Social Subjects. No. 18. (1980). *Artificial Feeds for the Young Infant. HMSO, London.*
15. American Academy of Pediatrics: Committee on Nutrition (1976). Commentary on breast feeding and infant formulas, including proposed standards for formulas. *Pediatrics* **57**, 278–85.
16. American Academy of Pediatrics: Committee on Nutrition (1977). Nutritional needs of low birth weight infants. *Pediatrics* **60**, 519–30.
17. Canadian Paediatric Society: Committee on Nutrition (1981). Feeding the low birth weight infant. *Can. Med. Ass.* **124**, 1301–11.
18. American Academy of Pediatrics: Committee on Nutrition (1985). Nutritional needs of low birthweight infants. *Pediatrics* **75**, 976–86.
19. Ganther H.E., Hafeman D.G., Lawrence R.A., Serfass R.E. & Hoeskstra W.E. (1976). Selenium and glutathione peroxidase in health and disease: review. In: *Trace Elements in Human Health and Disease* Vol. 1 (eds A.S. Prasad & D. Oberleas) pp165–237. Academic Press, New York.
20. Awasthi Y.C., Beutler E. & Srivastava S.K. (1975). Purification and properties of human erythrocyte glutathione peroxidase. *J. Biol. Chem.* **250**, 5144–9.
21. Schwartz K. (1965). Role of vitamin E, selenium, and related factors in experimental nutrtional liver disease. *Fed. Proc.* **24**, 58–67.
22. Westermarck T. (1977). Selenium content of tissues in Finnish infants and adults with various diseases, and studies on the effects of selenium supplementation in neuronal ceroid lipofuscinosis patients. *Acta Pharmacol. Toxicol.* **41**, 121–8.
23. Glader B.E. & Conrad M.E. (1972). Decreased glutathione peroxidase in neonatal erythrocytes: lack of relation to hydrogen peroxide metabolism. *Pediatr. Res.* **6**, 900–4.
24. Hågå P. & Lunde G. (1978). Selenium and vitamin E in cord blood from preterm and full term infants. *Acta Pediatr. Scand.* **67**, 235–9.
25. Lombeck I., Kasperek K., Harbisch H.D., Feinendegen L.E. & Bremer H.J. (1977). The selenium concentration at different ages; activity of glutathione peroxidase of erythrocytes at different ages; selenium content in food of infants. *Eur. J. Pediatr.* **125**, 81–8.
26. von Stockhausen H.B., Negretti V.E. & Bratter P. (1984). Spurenelement analysen bei Früh—und Neugeborenen sowie säuglingen unter einer parenteralen infusions therapie mit besonderer Berücksichtigung des Selens. *Mschr. Kinderheilk.* **132**, 727.
27. Smith A.M., Picciano M.F. & Milner J.A. (1982). Selenium intake and status of human milk and formula fed infants. *Am. J. Clin. Nutr.* **35**, 521–8.
28. Amin S., Chen S.Y., Collipp P.J., Castro-Magana M., Maddaiah V.T. & Klein S.W. (1980). Selenium in premature infants. *Nutr. Metab.* **24**, 331–40.
29. Musa Al-Zubaidi I., Lombeck I., Feinendegen L.E. & Bremer H.J. (1982). Hair selenium content during infancy and childhood. *Eur. J. Pediatr.* **139**, 295–6.
30. Lombeck I., Kasperek K., Bonnermann B., Feinendegen L.E. & Bremer H.J. (1978). Selenium content of human milk, cow's milk and cow's milk infant formulas. *Eur. J. Pediatr.* **129**, 139—45.
31. Higashi A., Tamari H., Kuroki Y. & Matsuda I. (1983). Longitudinal changes in selenium content of breast milk. *Acta Paediatr. Scand.* **72**, 433–6.

32. Chen X., Yang G., Chen J., Chen X., Wen Z. & Ge K. (1980). Studies on the relation of selenium and Keshan disease. *Biol. Trace Element Res.* **2**, 91–107.

33. Johnson R.A., Baker S.S., Fallon J.J., Maynard E.P., Ruskin J.N., Wen Z., Ge K. & Cohen A.J. (1981). An occidental case of cardiomyopathy and selenium deficiency *N. Engl. J. Med.* **304**, 1210–2.

34. King W.W.-K., Miche I.L., Wood W.C., Malt R.A., Baker S.S. & Cohen H.J. (1981). Reversal of selenium deficiency with oral selenium. *N. Engl. J. Med.* **304**, 1305.

35. Baker S.S., Lerman R.H., Krey S.H., Crocker K.S., Hirch E.F. & Cohen H. (1983). Selenium deficiency with total parenteral nutrition: Reversible biochemical and functional abnormalities by selenium supplementation: A case report. *Am. J. Clin. Nutr.* **38**, 769–74.

36. Lombeck I., Kasperek K., Harbisch H.D., Becker K., Schumann E., Schröter W., Feinendegen L.E. & Bremer H.J. (1978). The selenium state of children. II. Selenium content of serum, whole blood, hair and the activity of erythrocyte glutathione peroxidase in dietetically treated patients with phenylketonuria and maple syrup urine disease. *Eur. J. Pediatr.* **128**, 213–23.

37. Lombeck I., Kasperek K., Bachmann D., Feinendegen L.E. & Bremer H.J. (1980). Selenium requirements in patients with inborn errors of amino acid metabolism and selenium deficiency. *Eur. J. Pediatr.* **134**, 65–8.

38. Robberecht H., Roekens E. & Van Caille-Bertrand M. (1985). Longitudinal study of selenium content in human breast milk in Belgium. *Acta Paediatr. Scand.* **74**, 254–8.

39. Kumpulainen J., Vuori E., Kuitunen P., Makinen S. & Kara R (1983). Longitudinal study on the dietary selenium intake of exclusively breat fed infants and their mothers in Finland. *Int. J. Vit. Nutr. Res.* **53**, 420–6.

40. ESPGAN Committee on Nutrition: Guidelines on Infant Nutrition (1977). I. Recommendation for the Composition of an Adapted Formula. *Acta Paediatr. Scand.* (Suppl.) **262**.

41. Department of Health and Social Security (1980). Report on Health and Social Subjects. No. 18. Artificial Feeds for the Young Infant. HMSO, London.

42. American Academy of Pediatrics: Committee in Nutrition (1976). Commentary on breast feeding and infant formulas, including proposed standards for formulas. *Pediatrics* **57**, 278–85.

43. American Academy of Pediatrics: Committee on Nutrition (1977). Nutritional needs of low birth weight infants. *Pediatrics* **60**, 519–30.

44. Canadian Paediatric Society: Committee on Nutrition (1981). Feeding the low birth weight infant. *Can. Med. Ass.* **124**, 1301–11.

45. American Academy of Pediatrics: Committee on Nutrition (1985). Nutritional needs of low birthweight infants. *Pediatrics* **75**, 976–86.

46. Coughlan M.P. ed. (1980). *Molybdenum and Molybdenum-Containing Enzymes.* Pergamon Press, Oxford.

47. Coughlan M.P. (1983). The role of molybdenum in human biology. *J. Inherited. Metab. Dis.* **6**, (Suppl.) 70–7.

48. Johnson J.L., Hainelin B.E. & Rajagopalan K.V. (1980). Characterization of the molybdenum cofactor of sulfite oxidase. xanthine oxidase, and nitrate reductase: identification of a pteridine as a structural component. *J. Biol. Chem.* **255**, 1783–6.

49. Duran M., Beemer F.A., van de Heiden G., Korteland J., de Bree P.K., Brink M. & Wadman S.K. (1978). Combined deficiency of xanthine oxidase and sulfite oxidase: a effect of molybdenum metabolism or transport? *J. Inherited Met. Dis.* **1**, 175–8.

50. Johnson J.L., Wand W.R., Rajagopalan K.V., Duran M, Beemer F.A. & Wadman S.K. (1980). Inborn error of molybdenum metabolism: combined deficiencies of sulphite oxidase and xanthine dehydrogenase in a patient lacking the molybdenum cofactor. *Proc. Nat. Acad. Sci.* **77**, 3715–9.

51. Abumrad N.N., Schneider A.J., Steel D. & Rogers L.S. Amino acid intolerance during total parenteral nutrition reversed by molybdate therapy. *Am. J. Clin. Nutr.* **34**, 2551–9.

52. Archibald J.G. (1958). Trace elements in milk' A Review, Part II *Dairy Sci. Abst.* **20**, 800–12.
53. Antila P. (1973). Occurrence of certain trace elements in cows milk. *Finnish J. Dairy Sci.* **32**, 8–13.
54. Kirchgessner M., Friesecke H. & Koch G. (1967). *Nutrition and the Composition of Milk.* Crosby Lockwood & Son Ltd, London.
55. Mertz W. (1969). Chromium occurrence and function in biological systems. *Phys. Rev.* **49**, 163–239.
56. Mertz W., Toepfer E.W. & Rozinski E.E. (1974). Present knowledge of the role of chromium. *Fed. Proc.* **33**, 2275–80.
57. Anderson R.A. & Mertz W. (1977). Glucose tolerance factor: an essential dietary agent. *Trends Biol. Sci.* **2**, 277–9.
58. Shapcott D. & Hubat J., eds (1979). *Chromium in Nutrition and Metabolism.* Elsevier (North Holland) Biomedical Press, Amsterdam.
59. Wallach S. & Verch R.L. (1984). Plancental transport of chromium. *J. Am. Coll. Nutr.* **3**, 69–74.
60. Widdowson E.M., Chan H., Harrison G.E. & Milner R.D.G. (1972). Accumulation of Cu, Zn, Cr and Co in the human liver before birth. *Biol. Neonat.* **20**, 360–7.
61. Anderson R.A. & Polansky M.M. (1981). Dietary chromium deficiency. Effect on sperm count and fertility in rats. *Biol. Trace Elem. Res.* **3**, 1–5.
62. Mirsky N., Weiss A. & Dori Z. (1980). Chromium in biological systems. 1. Some observations on glucose tolerance factor in yeast. *J. Inorg. Biol.* **13**, 11–21.
63. Mirsky N., Weiss A. & Dori Z. (1981). The effect of glucose tolerance factor on glucose uptake by yeast cells. *J. Inorg. Biochem.* **15**, 275–9.
64. Haylock S.J., Buckley P.D. & Blackwell L.F. (1983). Separation of biologically active chromium-containing complexes from yeast extracts and other sources of glucose tolerance factor (GTF) activity. *J. Inorg. Biochem.* **18**, 195–211.
65. Haylock S.J., Buckley P.D. & Blackwell L.F. (1983). The relationship of chromium to the glucose tolerance factor II. *J. Inorg. Biochem.* **19**, 105–17.
66. Jeeejeeboy K.N., Chu R.C., Marliss E.B., Greenberg G.R. & Bruce-Robertson A. (1977). Chromium deficiency, glucose intolerance and neuropathy reversed by chromium supplementation in a patient receiving long term total parenteral nutrition. *Am. J. Clin. Nutr.* **30**, 531–8.
67. Freund H., Atamian S. & Fischer J.E. (1979). Chromium deficiency during total parenteral nutrition. *J. Am. Med. Assoc.* **241**, 496–8.
68. Kumpulainen J. & Vuori E. (1980). Longitudinal study of chromium in human milk. *Am. J. Clin. Nutr.* **33**, 2299–302.
69. Pharoah P.O.D., Buttfield I.H. & Hetzel B.S. (1971). Neurological damage to the fetus resulting in severe iodine deficiency during pregnancy. *Lancet* **i**, 308–10.
70. Delange F., Ermans A.M., Vis H.L. & Stanbury J.B. (1972). Endemic cretinism in Idjwi Island (Kivu Lake, Republic of the Congo). *J. Clin. Endocr. Metab.* **34**, 1059–66.
71. Delange F., Bourdoux P., Ketelbant-Balasse P., Van Humskerken A., Glinoer D. & Ermans A.M. (1983). Transient primary hypothyroidism in the newborn. In: *Congenital hypothyroidism,* (eds J.H. Dussault & P. Walker) pp. 275–301 M. Dekker, New York.
72. Salter W.T., (1950). The chemistry and physiology of the thryroid horome. In: *The Hormones: Physiology, Chemistry and Applications,* (eds G. Pincus & K.V. Thiman) Vol. 2. Academic Press, New York.
73. Department of Health and Social Security (1980). Artificial feeds for the young infant. Report on Health and Social Subjects 18. HMSO, London.
74. Hurley L.S. (1980). *Developmental Nutrition.* Prentice & Hall, Englewood Cliffs, New Jersey.
75. Dodd F.H., Kingwell R.G., Shearn M.F.H., Morant S.V. & Lewis G. (1975). Iodine levels in milk following iodophor teat disinfection. National Institute for Research in Dairying, Report

1973–4. p. 57.
76. Backer Dirks O., Jongeling-Eijndhoven J., Flissebaalje T. *et al.* 91974). Total and free ionic fluoride in human and cows milk as determined by gas-liquid chromatography and the fluoride electrode. *Caries Res.* **8**, 181.

14
The Effect of Dietary Composition on Whole Body Net Base Balance

INTRODUCTION

The pH of the plasma and extracellular fluid is determined by the concentration and chemical characteristics of the dissolved acids and bases. In health the concentration of the different acids and bases in the ECF are controlled such that the pH is maintained within the range 7.36–7.45 (35–44 nmol/l). In preterm infants acidosis of some degree invariably occurs at the time of birth and results from the hypoxia and carbon dioxide retention associated with the birth process and the transition to pulmonary ventilation. However, disturbances of plasma pH occurring after the first week of life are also common and in a number of instances have been shown to be related to the composition of the diet; it is these disturbances of pH that are the subject of this chapter. During growth the fetus, infant and child are all in positive base balance, and the majority of the base is deposited in the skeleton. Most of this base is provided by the diet and it is essential therefore, if acid base disturbances are to be avoided, to pay careful attention to the composition of the diet. This is particularly important for the preterm infants as their renal tubular mechanisms responsible for the maintenance of base balance are immature and are easily overcharged.

The first measurements of base balance in infants were made by Shohl & Sato (1924) (1). Subsequently Relman and his colleagues using a slightly different approach drew attention to the role of diet composition on the balance of net acid (2–6). More recently Kildeberg has further developed the concepts of acid base physiology and in particular the concept of net base balance (7,8). What follows is a compressed account of the concepts developed by Kildeberg (7), which it is hoped will serve as an introduction to the subject. The reader is strongly recommended to read his most recent work. Much of the difficulty of this subject is due to the ambiguity and unfamiliarity of the terms used, so if this chapter is to be understood it is necessary to begin with some definitions.

TERMINOLOGY

An acid is defined as a molecule or ion that under certain conditions can dissociate to yield a hydrogen ion (proton) and its conjugate base.

$$H_2B \rightleftharpoons H^+ + HB^- \rightleftharpoons 2H^+ + B^{2-} \qquad [1]$$

Conversely a base is a molecule or ion that can under certain circumstances accept a hydrogen ion.

In acid base chemistry it is necessary to define the amount of an acid by quantifying the property by which it is defined, that is the extent to which the above reaction has proceeded from left to right. Thus the amount of acid present in a solution is defined as the amount of hydrogen ions donated and this is commonly measured by back titration with a strong base. However, the amount of hydrogen ions donated depends not only on the concentration and pK of the acids and bases, but also on the pH, temperature, and ionic strength of the solution. Therefore in practice the amount of acid present in a solution is measured by titration to an arbitrarily chosen endpoint or reference state defined by the pH, temperature and ionic strength of the solution. With respect to blood plasma the appropriate reference state is defined as pH 7.4, temp 37°C and ionic strength 0.17 mol/kg H_2O. It follows from this that in the reference state the amount of titratable acid (TA) for example in plasma is by definition equal to zero.

In the discussion that follows A stands for acid and B for base, the prefix c stands for concentration, t for the total amount of a substance and the suffix u for urine. A sign convention governs the terms A and B such that $-cTA = cTB$ and vice versa. Square brackets enclosing symbols refer to the rate of intake, absorption, excretion, or retention for the whole body of the substance in mmol/kg per day.

KINDS OF ACID

There are three kinds of acid in the body.

Carbonic acid (CA)

Carbonic acid is formed by the hydration of carbon dioxide and it dissociates into bicarbonate and carbonate ions thus:

$$CO_2 + H_2O \rightleftharpoons H_2CO_3 \rightleftharpoons H^+ + HCO_3^- \rightleftharpoons 2H^+ + CO_3^{2-} \qquad [2]$$

In accordance with the definition of the *amount* of acid given above the concentration of carbonic acid (cCA) is defined as being equal to the extent (per unit volume) that the reaction in equation [2] has proceeded from left to right. However, since all hydrogen ions are alike the amount of hydrogen ions donated can only be determined from the concentration of the conjugate bases multiplying by the number of negative charges on each of them. Hence the cCA is equal to the sum of the $cHCO_3^- + 2(cCO_3^{2-})$, which from the Henderson-Hasselbalch equation (with pK_{A1} of 6.1 and pK_{A2} of 10.2) can be shown to be equal to 0.9538 $(ctCO_2)$ in the reference state (pH 7.4, temperature 37°C, and ionic strength 0.17 mol/kg H_2O). The cCA in the plasma is maintained at about 24 mmol/l. It is controlled by pulmonary ventilation and cannot be primarily influenced by changes in diet. However, in response to changes in the concentration of other acids or bases in the blood (see below) compensatory changes in alveolar ventilation may cause the cCA to rise or fall in order to return the plasma pH towards normal.

Non-carbonic acid (NCA)

NCA is titratable acid comprising acids and bases other than carbonic acid. There are two kinds of non-carbonic acid in the body.

Metabolizable acid (MA)

MA is titratable acid or base made up of organic acids and bases which are either absorbed from the diet or formed in the course of tissue metabolism which can be disposed of by intermediary metabolism. They may be quite simple organic acids for example:

$$\text{Glucose} \rightarrow 2 \text{ lactate} + 2 H^+ + 6 O_2 \rightarrow 6 CO_2 + 6 H_2O \qquad [3]$$

or they may consist of metabolizable acid and base groups on much larger molecules such as proteins. In the steady state in the normal individual the sum of the rate of absorption and production of MA is equal to its rate of removal by intermediary metabolism, and rate of excretion in the urine. The cMA in the body is controlled by the metabolic processes responsible for the turnover of MA and in ordinary circumstances is little influenced by variations in the amount of MA in the diet. The cMA in the plasma for example is relatively constant and amounts to about 17 mmol/l of which about 65% is protein.

Though MA is excreted in the urine the amount present in the body is not under renal control.

Non-metabolizable acid (net acid or net base) (NA, NB)

NA is a titratable acid ($cNA = -cNB$) consisting of acids and bases that cannot be disposed of by intermediary metabolism or by pulmonary ventilation. They may be absorbed from the diet, or formed within the body as end products of irreversible metabolic processes such as the oxidation of inorganic sulphur in sulphur containing amino acids to sulphuric acid.

$$Methionine + O_2 \rightarrow Urea + CO_2 + H_2O + SO_4^{2-} + 2H^+ \qquad [4]$$

Other non-metabolizable end products of metabolism such as creatinine, uric acid, bilirubin and taurine also contribute to NA, but are quantitatively of so little importance that they cannot be ignored (7). The principal acids and bases are sodium hydroxide, potassium hydroxide, calcium hydroxide, magnesium hydroxide, hydrochloric acid, phosphoric acid, and sulphuric acid.

These acids and bases exist in different combinations in different tissues, but using blood plasma as an example will make the nature of non-metabolizable acid clear. The acids and bases mentioned above can be considered to be stochiometrically present in plasma at all times but, because they react with each other and with other plasma constituents (MA and CA), the amount of each acid or base stochiometrically present can only be estimated from the concentration of its associated non-metabolizable anion (in the case of an acid) or non-metabolizable cation (in the case of a base). Since the concentration of the non-metabolizable cations in plasma exceeds the concentration of the non-metabolizable anions, plasma contains a negative concentration of NA, that is a positive concentration of NB.

The cNB in plasma (or in diet, stool or urine) can in principle be defined as the concentration of titratable acid on titration to the reference state (see above) *when cCA and cMA are both zero*. However, this is not possible in practice because the NB of plasma is fully titrated with CA and MA. Therefore operationally the concentration of NB is determined as the difference between the sum of the non-metabolizable cations and the sum of the non-metabolizable anions multiplying by the value of the average positive or negative charge present in the reference state. The following general equation relates the concentration of NB to the concentration of the non-metabolizable ions in the reference state, and can be applied to any biological medium.

$$cNB = (cNa^+ + cK^+ + 2cCa^{2+} + 2cMg^{2+}) \quad [5]$$
$$- (cCl^- + 2ctSO_4^{2-} + 1.8ctP)$$

Note that 1.8 is the average negative charge per mole of phosphate at pH 7.4 measured as total (oxidized) phosphorus represented by the symbol tP. From the buffer equation

$$pH = pK + \log \frac{(HPO_4^{2-})}{(H_2PO_4^-)} \qquad [pK = 6.8.] \qquad [6]$$

it can be shown that one mole of phosphoric acid dissociates at pH 7.4 to yield 0.8 HPO_4^{2-} and 0.2 $H_2PO_4^-$, i.e. $(2 \times 0.8) + 0.2 = 1.8$.

From equation [5] it can be shown that plasma has a cNB of about 41 mmol/1. Since the concentration of TA in the reference state is by definition zero, then:

$$cMA + cCA - cNB = cTA \qquad [7]$$
$$= 0$$

Substituting the values given above for the concentration of the different kinds of acid in plasma $17 + 24 - 41 = 0$ and the cNCA is -24mmol/1. The concentration of NB in the plasma is under specific renal control and in the normal steady state is equal to the sum of the cCA and cMA. In practice it is not possible to measure the cMA and it is therefore determined from equation [7] where cMA = cTA − cCA + cNB. Since cTA − cCA = cNCA then the cMA is equal to cNCA + cNB.

WHOLE BODY NB BALANCE

Since the principal source of NB is the absorbed products of digestion of the diet, and the only route of excretion is in the urine it is possible using standard metabolic balance techniques to determine the whole body balance of NB; one cannot derive balances for MA and CA as it is not possible to measure input of these acids independently of output. An understanding of the whole body NB balance is important for two reasons. In the first place the growing infant and child is in a positive balance for NB, most of which is laid down in the skeleton, and the diet is the principal source of this base. Secondly, because the capacity of the kidney of the preterm infant to secrete hydrogen ions is limited, variations in the NB of the diet that might be of no significance to a more mature infant can produce serious changes in the cNB of the plasma and metabolic acidosis.

The balance of net base is defined by the following equations:

$$[NB\ Balance] = [NB\ Input] - [NB\ Output] \tag{8}$$

$$[NB\ Input] = [NB\ Diet] - [NB\ Stool] \tag{9}$$

$$[NB\ Output] = [NB\ Urine] \tag{10}$$

The NB of the diet and stool and urine is estimated by using equation [5], after chemical analysis of the inorganic components. It is, however, necessary to omit the analysis of sulphate (in diet and stool) from the input expression of the balance equation. The reason for this is that with a well balanced diet the majority of the sulphur containing amino acids will be incorporated into new body tissue during growth and only small amounts of sulphur will be oxidized to sulphuric acid (see equation [4]). However, in the ashing process that is a necessary preliminary to chemical analysis, all the sulphur will be oxidized to sulphuric acid and the inclusion of total sulphate would result in an overestimate of sulphuric acid production. In the healthy growing infant zero sulphate balance is assumed to obtain so the amount of sulphate present in the urine each day (output) is presumed to represent all the sulphate produced by oxidation of sulphur in sulphur containing amino acids (input). It is this amount that should be included in the input expression of the balance equation. If sulphate were omitted from both the input and output (urine) expressions of the balance equation there would be no error in the estimate of the NB balance, but the NB of the urine would be overestimated, and the effect of excess amounts of sulphur containing amino acids in the diet might be over-looked.

Changes in non-metabolizable base during fetal growth and the effect of skeletal mineralization

From equation [10] and using the results of chemical analyses of fetal bodies it is possible to calculate the change in the concentration of NB of the fetus during growth. According to Kildeberg (1981) (7) the fetal NB rises from 140 mmol/kg at 23 weeks gestation to 238 mmol/kg at 35 weeks gestation. This positive NB balance arises mainly from the incorporation of base into the hydroxyapatite mineral of bone. For example:

$$10Ca^{2+} + 4.8HPO_4^{2-} + 1.2H_2PO_4^- + 2H_2O \rightleftharpoons$$
$$(Ca_3(PO_4)_2)_3 \cdot Ca(OH)_2 + 9.2H^+ \qquad [11]$$

Thus for each mmol of calcium laid down in the hydroxyapatite of bone 0.92 mmol of base is bound and 0.92 mmolH$^+$ are released into the ECF. According to Kildeberg *et al.* (1969) (9) direct titration of bone gives a rather lower value and they used 0.8 mmol H$^+$/mmol Ca^{2+}. From estimates of the accumulation of calcium *in utero* by the human fetus it can be calculated that the skeleton binds between 2.4–3.1 mmol NB/kg per day which must be provided by placental transfer of NB. If an intrauterine rate of skeletal mineralization is to take place in a preterm infant the NB would have to be absorbed from the diet since the mechanisms for renal NB regeneration would be insufficient (see below).

Non-metabolizable base of milk

Table 14.1 gives estimates of the NB of some milks used for infant feeding and

Table 14.1. (a) Estimate of the non-metabolizable base content of different milks and the daily intake at the recommended volumes.

MILK	VOL ml/kg per day	Na	K	Ca	Mg (mmol/1)	P	CC	NB	NB mmol/ kg per day
Cow milk	180	22.0	38.0	30.0	5.00	31.0	27.0	47.2	8.5
Breast milk (early)	200	21.0	17.0	6.3	0.85	5.2	24.0	18.9	3.8
Breast milk (mature)	200	6.0	15.0	8.5	1.25	4.5	12.0	20.4	4.1
Full term formula	200	6.5	14.4	11.0	2.20	10.6	10.4	17.8	3.6
Preterm formulae									
A	150	14.0	19.2	19.0	2.90	13.0	14.9	38.7	5.8
B	180	8.7	15.4	25.0	6.25	16.1	11.3	46.4	8.3
C	150	26.1	24.4	16.8	4.58	17.1	22.5	39.8	6.0
D	180	19.6	16.7	17.5	2.10	11.3	16.9	38.2	6.9
Soy formula	180	9.0	19.0	16.0	2.85	14.3	11.0	29.0	5.2

(**b**) Amounts of different kinds of acid in milk and pH (7).

	cCA	cMA	cNB (mmol/1)	cTA	pH
Human milk	4.9	23.0	22.0	5.9	6.6
Cow milk	4.1	61.0	55.0	10.1	6.5

also estimates of the different kinds of acids in human and cow's milk (7). The cNB is variable being highest in cow's milk and preterm formulae and lowest in human milk and adapted formulae designed for full term infants. Nevertheless the intake of NB from any of the milks in Table 14.1 is more than sufficient to neutralize all the acid produced from bone mineralization and other sources but not all of it is absorbed. The positive cTA of the milks is due to the excess of (cCA + cMA) over cNB, but since these acids are readily disposed of in ordinary circumstances by pulmonary ventilation and intermediary metabolism they are not likely to contribute to the acidosis of dietary origin seen in preterm infants.

Absorption of non-metabolizable base by preterm infants

Kildeberg *et al.* (1969) (9) studying eight low birth-weight infants fed a partially adapted full term formula showed that with of an average NB intake of 7.1 mmol/kg per day only 0.5 mmol/kg per day was absorbed, the remainder appearing in the stools. The NB absorption was close to the NB estimated to be laid down in the skeleton over the same period of time namely 0.57 mmol/kg per day. In contrast two infants fed cow's milk had a mean NB intake of 12.4 mmol/kg per day and absorbed 1.51 mmol/kg per day and this served to furnish the NB for skeletal mineralization which averaged 1.53 mmol/kg per day. There seems therefore to be a close approximation between the [NB] absorption and the rate of deposition of NB in the developing skeleton. These data may have underestimated the NB absorption (Kildeberg, personal communication). Studies of full term infants (10) and of weanling rats (11) suggest that NB absorption in growing young may be as high as 40% of intake. It is important to emphasize that since the majority of the dietary sodium, potassium, magnesium, chloride and phosphate are absorbed, the absorbed NB depends very much on the calcium absorption. This means that on a diet of given composition variations in calcium absorption and skeletal mineraliz-ation, because they are associated with parallel changes in NB absorption, will not alter the NB balance. However, an increase in calcium absorption and bone deposition will utilize some of the absorbed phosphate and urinary phosphate would therefore be reduced. This in its turn would reduce the urinary buffer capacity.

Balance of non-metabolizable base in growing infants

It is unfortunate that there are no published data on the NA excretion in the urine of preterm infants. However, Kildeberg *et al.* (1969) (9) found that preterm infants weighing 1.2–2.0 kg were in positive NB balance averaging +1.0 mmol/day and 1–2 month old full term infants fed cow's milk were in positive NB balance averaging +1.37 mmol/kg per day (8). The retained base was provided almost entirely by absorbed base from the diet and the positive $[NA]_{urine}$ (see equation [5]) was mainly due to the metabolism of sulphur containing amino acids to yield small amounts of sulphuric acid.

Renal mechanisms for the control of non-metabolizable base balance

The concentrations of NB, CA, and MA in the glomerular filtrate are 35, 26, and 9 mmol/l respectively (7) and the TA is close to zero. The amount of NB filtered is dependent on the product of the plasma concentration and the GFR, and though it will change with changes in GFR the process is essentially non-selective depending on the plasma concentration.

The majority of the filtered NB (about 75%) is reabsorbed together with CA (as HCO_3^-) by controlled and selective tubular mechanisms which determine the plasma NB concentration. In the renal tubular cell CO_2 is rapidly hydrated in the presence of carbonic anhydrase and water to form H_2CO_3 which dissociates into H^+ and HCO_3^-. The H^+ is transported into the tubular lumen in exchange for sodium ions, and the HCO_3^- (i.e. $OH^- + CO_2$ together with Na^+) is returned to the circulation thus regenerating the filtered NB (10).

The remaining 25% of the filtered NB is present in the filtrate as the salts of MA (e.g. $R-COO^- + Na^+$). A proportion of the organic anion is reabsorbed together with non-metabolizable cations (e.g. Na^+), but the remainder of the organic anion appears in the urine. Since the pK of the organic acids of these anions are below the minimum urinary pH attainable by preterm infants probably less than 10% can be excreted as free acids, and if the remainder were excreted as the salts of the acids a significant amount of the filtered NB would be lost in the urine, and NB regeneration would be incomplete. What appears to happen is that as the NB is regenerated and hydrogen ions are secreted into the tubular lumen some of the MA is neutralized by the strong base NH_3 (pK 9.3) secreted by the renal tubules and the remainder is buffered by phosphate. In the body the regenerated NB may react irreversibly to neutralize metabolizable acid.

The H^+ ions secreted into the tubular lumen thus take part in four main reactions. The majority (about 75%) react with luminal HCO_3^- to produce CO_2 and water. The remaining H^+ ions titrate the HPO_4^{2-} to $H_2PO_4^-$ and $R-COO^-$ to $R-COOH$. However, the extent of these two latter reactions depend on the pK of the bases involved and the minimum attainable pH of the urine (see below). If the pH falls too low the H^+ ion pump is blocked. Under these circumstances the NH_3 generation increases, effectively eliminating H^+ ions and permitting their continued secretion.

The rate of renal NB regeneration (tubular H^+ secretion) is normally regulated to maintain a plasma cNB that is equal to the sum of the cMA and cCA, but the mechanism by which it is controlled is at present poorly understood. It is evident that the plasma NB *concentration* is determined by the net gains and losses by the ECF of both NB and water but if the *amount* of NB in the ECF is to remain constant, the rate of tubular NB regeneration ($[NB]_{tr}$) must be equal to the difference between the NB filtered ($[NB]_f$) and the NB entering the ECF from other sources such as gastrointestinal absorption, parenteral infusion, skeletal mineralization or intracellular metabolism ($[NB_{ECF}]_{in}$). Also if the NB balance of the ECF is to remain zero then the $[NB_{ECF}]_{in}$ must be equal to the NB present in the urine ($[NB]_u$). In the steady state therefore:

$$[NB_{ECF}]_{in} = [NB]_f - [NB]_{tr} = [NB]_u \qquad [12]$$

If the maximum rate of tubular NB reabsorption is limited then the $[NB]_u$ will exceed the $[NB_{ECF}]_{in}$ and the plasma NB concentration will fall and a metabolic acidosis will develop. The fall in cNB will lead to a fall in the $[NB]_f$ until a new steady state is reached (equation [12]).

From the foregoing it is clear that the $[NB]_u$ must be the difference between the filtered base and the tubular hydrogen ion secretion. The $[NB]_u$ is generally negative, i.e. a positive $[NA]_u$. It can be expressed in two ways, by equation [5] given above and by the following equation:

$$[NA]_u = [TA']_u + [NH_4^+]_u - [R\text{-}COO^-]_u \qquad [13]$$

where $[TA']_u$ is the amount of titratable acid in the urine after titration to pH 7.4 at a PCO_2 of 0 mmHg and $[R\text{-}COO^-]$ is the amount of filtered metabolizable anion in the urine following titration of the urine to pH 7.4. Expressed in this way the $[NA]_u$ is shown to be equal to the difference between the filtered base and the tubular secretion of hydrogen ions (7). From equation [13] it can be seen that the NA in the urine is not only affected by the capacity for the tubules to secrete hydrogen ions but also by the amount of filtered base, and the amount that is reabsorbed.

It should be noted that equations [5] & [13] differ fundamentally from the earlier definitions of Net Acid Excretion used by Relman and his colleagues (2–6). (For a full discussion see references 7 and 8.)

Renal tubular function in preterm infants

Studies of preterm infants aged 2–3 weeks have shown that their urine contains both titratable acid and ammonia and that both increase in response to NA loading with NH_4Cl. However, compared with full term infants $[TA]_u$ and

$[NH_4^+]_u$ increased to only 57% and 43% of the maximum values observed in full term infants (13). This diminished capacity to increase tubular hydrogen ion secretion and therefore NB regeneration is a major determinant of late metabolic acidosis (see below). By 4–6 weeks when the acidosis has generally disappeared, the maximal TA_u and $NH_4^+{}_u$ are comparable to those seen in full term infants (13). If the tubular NB regeneration is limited by immaturity of tubular function then the amount of filtered and unreabsorbed base becomes an important determinant of the NB concentration of the blood.

Filtered and unreabsorbed base

The data of Kildeberg *et al.* (1969) (9) from preterm infants showed that the $(TA'_u + NH_4^+{}_u)$ averaged 2.85 mmol/day and the urinary titratable organic anion averaged 2.24 mmol/day. The difference of 0.61 mmol/day, which approximates the NA of the urine (see equations [5] & [13], was mainly accounted for by the sulphuric acid production as the urinary sulphate ($2SO_4^{2-}$) averaged 0.35 mmol/day. It thus would appear that in preterm infants much of the renal tubular hydrogen ion secretion (of which more than half is NH_4^+ and the remainder is titratable acid) is consequent on the reabsorption of NB filtered with MA. As has been pointed out above the metabolizable acids have pK values for the most part below the minimum urinary pH attainable by preterm infants so the passage of large amounts of organic anion in the urine may necessitate either a higher buffer capacity of the urine (see below) or an increased secretion of NH_3. However, as the amount of buffer in the urine is not under the infants control and the capacity to increase NH_3 secretion is limited, the filtered and unreabsorbed organic anion may indirectly, by preventing NB reabsorption, cause loss of NB in the urine and metabolic acidosis.

There is little quantitative or qualitative information on the organic acids in the urine of preterm infants, or on the effect of diet composition on their rate of excretion. Nevertheless, the presence of such high concentrations of organic anion in the urine is probably due to decreased tubular absorption reflecting the general level of immaturity of renal function.

It is worth pointing out here that in situations where very large amounts of MA are produced (e.g. lactic acidosis due to tissue hypoxia, or diabetic ketoacidosis) substantial amounts of MA appear in the urine. If these circumstances persist for any length of time the capacity of the tubules to secrete hydrogen ions and hence reabsorb NB may be overcharged and large amounts of NB can be lost in the urine. This has the effect of converting the lactic acidosis in part into an NA acidosis (or NB subtraction acidosis).

Urinary phosphate and buffer value

Because phosphate (pK 6.8) is the principal buffer in urine it is essential that there is sufficient in the urine to allow tubular hydrogen ion secretion to proceed within the limits set by the minimum urinary pH (about pH 5.0–5.6 (14)) and the capacity of the kidney to generate ammonia. Using the buffer equation (equation [6]) it can be shown that 1.0 mmol phosphate titrated from pH 7.4 to pH 5.6 would buffer 0.74 mmol H^+. The $[TA']_u$ is very unlikely to exceed that seen in infants fed cow's milk, about 1.9 mmol/kg per day (9) which would require not more than 2.5 mmol P/kg per day. Infants fed partially adapted full term formulae are reported to have a $[TA']_u$ of about 1.04 mmol/kg per day which would require a maximum of 1.4 mmol P/kg per day. However, the single infant whose complete data is given by Kildeberg *et al.* (1969) (9) passed 1.09 mmol P/kg per day in his urine which would have titrated a maximum of only 0.8 mmol H^+/kg per day at pH 5.6. In fact the $[TA']_u$ was 1.07 mmol/kg per. day showing that phosphate was not the only buffer in the urine, and that phosphate can be less than the theoretical maximum.

In the present state of knowledge it is not possible to make firm recommendations about how much phosphate there should be in the urine, indeed the amount required depends very much on the composition of the diet and its effect on the whole body balance of NB which can only be determined by measurement. However, since the urinary phosphate is dependent on the dietary phosphate, the buffer value of the urine can be manipulated by varying the phosphate intake, but the effect of augmenting the dietary phosphate will depend on the form in which it is given.

The effect of dietary phosphate on NB balance

Phosphate may have different effects on NB balance depending on the form in which it is added to the diet. A neutral phosphate solution made up in a molar ratio of $4HPO_4^{2-}:1H_2PO_4^-$ has pH of 7.4. and an NB of zero. Supplementing with this mixture would have no effect on absorbed NB provided that the phosphate and its cation (e.g. sodium or potassium) were both absorbed to the same extent. However, there would be an increase in urinary phosphate buffer capacity and $[TA']_u$ would increase and the blood buffer base would shift towards zero if the infant was acidotic. Administering an acid phosphate salt such as NaH_2PO_4 which has a positive NA (0.8 mmol/mmol) would reduce the absorbed NB and might increase metabolic acidosis. If on the other hand, phosphate was present as a basic phosphate salt such as Na_2HPO_4 (NB = + 0.2 mmol/mmol) the absorbed NB, the $[NB]_u$ and the urinary phosphate would all be increased. If the phosphate was added as an organic phosphoester such as casein, the effect on the absorbed NB would depend on the NB of the casein preparation which depends on the method of preparation and degree of purification.

THE EFFECT OF DIET COMPOSITION ON ACID-BASE STATUS OF THE BLOOD

Late metabolic acidosis

Kildeberg (1964) (15) showed that preterm infants fed cow's milk formulae developed a late metabolic acidosis between one and three weeks after birth and he proposed that its cause was a disproportion between the daily load of 'non volatile acid' (NCA) generated in the body and the kidneys ability to excrete it. The late metabolic acidosis was characteristically more severe in infants fed high protein diets (15,16) and its incidence has been shown to vary directly with the protein intake (17,18). The acidosis which is often associated with a slow or absent weight gain responds to a temporary interruption of oral feeding and to sodium bicarbonate administration. However, while some have found that correction of the acidosis with bicarbonate increases weight gain (19) others have not (20).

It is axiomatic that during the development of metabolic acidosis NCA (i.e. MA-NB) input into the ECF must exceed NCA output until a new steady state is reached. However, the causes of late metabolic acidosis have not been systematically studied using the techniques outlined above, but such evidence as there is tends to show that negative NB balance is the principal determinant of late metabolic acidosis. Failure of the renal tubules to reabsorb organic anion may by the mechanisms given above contribute to the negative NB balance but it does not seem that excess production of MA is a major factor.

Table 14.2 gives the results of acid base studies in infants fed breast milk, a partially adapted full term formula and a half skimmed cow's milk (21). In the breast-fed infants there was no acidosis, the urine pH was above its minimum value and the $[TA]_u$, $[NH_4]_u$, and phosphate were the lowest of the three groups studied. The reverse was the case in the infants fed cow's milk. The value and the $[TA]_u$, $[NH_4]_u$, and phosphate were the lowest of the three data of Kildeberg *et al.* (1969) (9) were similar in that the $[SO_4^{2-}]_u$ in infants fed cow's milk (0.45 mmol/kg. per day) was four times the $[SO_4^{2-}]_u$ in infants fed a partially adapted full term formula (0.11 mmol/kg per day). Though there is insufficient data to calculate the $[NB]_u$ it is possible to derive approximate values. Using estimates for the $[Mg^{2+}]_u$ and $[SO_4^{2-}]_u$ the $[NB]_u$ of the breast-fed infants was $+0.81$ mmol/kg per day. On the adapted formula the estimated $[NB]_u$ was -0.74 mmol/kg per day (i.e. a positive $[NA]_u$) and on cow's milk the estimated $[NB]_u$ was -1.3 mmol/kg per day (also a positive $[NA]_u$)

Table 14.2. Acid base measurements in the plasma and urine of preterm infants fed different milks (21).

	Breast milk	Partially adapted full term formula	Half-skimmed cows milk
PLASMA			
pH	7.38 ±0.03	7.36 ±0.04	7.33 ±0.05
$PaCO_2$ mmHg	44.1 ±6.5	40.5 ±5.4	37.9 ±5.6
BE mmol/l	+0.1 ±1.6	−2.7 ±3.9	−5.5 ±3.21
URINE			
pH	6.05 ±0.57	5.72 ±0.45	5.30 ±0.44
mmol/kg per day			
$[TA]_u$	0.18 ±0.09	1.04 ±0.30	1.89 ±0.36
$[NH_4^+]_u$	0.64 ±0.22	1.31 ±0.32	1.63 ±0.41
$[Na^+]_u$	0.77 ±0.54	1.04 ?0.63	1.93 ±0.67
$[K^+]_u$	1.39 ±0.25	1.27 ±0.46	4.02 ±0.57
$[Ca^{2+}]_u$	0.25 ±0.13	0.07 ±0.04	0.05 ±0.03
$[Cl^-]_u$	1.45 ±0.57	1.47 ±0.55	3.91 ±0.53
$1.8[tP]_u$	0.03 ±0.02	1.19 ±0.32	2.18 ±0.32
$[SO_4^{2-}]_u$	0.43 ±0.09	0.59 ±0.20	1.32 ±0.21★

★Sulphate was estimated from the urinary nitrogen excretion and sulphur containing amino acid content of the diet(21).

These data show that late metabolic acidosis in preterm infants fed cow's milk probably develops because the rate of production of sulphuric acid from sulphur containing amino acids exceeds the rate at which NA can be excreted in the urine. This results in a loss of NB in the urine and the development of a metabolic acidosis. The few measurements of organic acids in the urine of preterm infants fed cow's milk or partially adapted formulae (9) suggest that the increased loss of organic anion in the urine may also be a significant factor in the development of the late metabolic acidosis of preterm infants.

Acidosis associated with acidified milks

Preterm infants fed half-cream cow's milk acidified with lactic or citric acid have been observed to develop a more severe acidosis than infants fed non-acidified milk (22). This was not due to the increase in MA in the diet since they excreted minute amounts of citric and lactic acid in the urine. It was thought to be due to a decrease in the [NB] absorption associated with an increased phosphate absorption. However, no change in NB absorption was observed in infants fed an acidified whey predominant formula, because the phosphate concentration was lower and the absorption high, so that no increase was possible (22).

Acidosis due to Nutramigen

Acidosis was reported in infants fed an earlier formulation of Nutramigen (23,24). Because no measurements of NB absorption, and urinary organic anion and sulphate excretion were made, the cause was never satisfactorily established but it seems likely that the low NB (16.5 mmol/1) played a part (25).

Alkalosis due to chloride deficient milk

Chloride deficiency due to both chloride deficient breast milk (26) and chloride deficient formulae have been described (27,28) (see p. 113). In these patients alkalosis was a prominent feature. It is thought that in the absence of sufficient chloride in the diet the demands of volume regulation cause an increase in the rate of tubular HCO_3^- regeneration to accompany the reabsorption of sodium ions. However, in part the alkalosis may have been due to volume contradiction (7).

THE EFFECT OF THE RECOMMENDATIONS ON THE NB OF THE DIET

Table 14.3 contains calculations based on the recommendations of this committee, but it is not intended to be a set of recommendations. It is purely a theoretical exercise to show how our recommendations might affect the NB of a preterm formula.

Table 14.3. Calculation of non-metabolizable base of a hypothetical formula based on the recommendations of this committee, and estimates of non-metabolizable base absorption.

Suggested requirements (at 130 kcal/kg per day)		Coefficient of absorption *
Na^+	1.3 –3.0 mmol/kg per day	0.8 –0.9
K^+	3.0 –5.0 mmol/kg per day	0.72–0.8
Ca^{2+}	2.3 –4.5 mmol/kg per day	0.6 –0.4
Mg^{2+}	0.33–0.65 mmol/kg per day	0.45
P	2.1 –3.7 mmol/kg per day	0.9
Cl^-	2.1 –3.3 mmol/kg per day	0.99

Estimated Dietary NB (see equation [5])
On minimum intakes = 3.64 mmol/kg per day (180 ml/kg per day = 20.2 mmol/l)
On maximum intakes = 8.30 mmol/kg per day (180 ml/kg per day = 46.1 mmol/l)

Estimate of Absorbed NB:
On minimum intakes = 0.75 mmol/kg per day (20% absorption)
On maximum intakes = 1.59 mmol/kg per day (19% absorption)

* Where a range is given the first value is the coefficient of absorption at minimum intake and the second is at maximum intake

Though these calculations of absorbed NB are only estimates, they fall within the range indicated in the Table 14.1 and would furnish sufficient NB for the likely rate of skeletal mineralization. There might not, however, be sufficient NB to neutralize the sulphuric acid production. If this were the case then the NB could be adjusted with sodium citrate (3.0 mmolNB/mmol). The ideal diet is probably one that would result in a $[NA]_u$ as close to zero as possible. Such a diet cannot be designed entirely on the drawing board, and the best composition will have to be found out by experiment. In particular the relationship between diet composition and the excretion of organic anion in the urine needs to be investigated.

CONCLUSIONS

1. Though milks may have a low pH and a measurable titratable acidity these H^+ ions usually make an insignificant contribution to the acidosis seen in preterm infants.
2. Milks should have a positive non-metabolizable base in appropriate concentration. The absorbed NB should be sufficient to provide the base for the observed rate of skeletal mineralization and also to neutralize the sulphuric acid produced from the breakdown of sulphur containing amino acids.
3. There should be sufficient sulphur containing amino acids in the diet to

satisfy the demands of growth but not so much that the production of sulphuric acid is excessive.

4. There should be sufficient phosphate in the diet to provide enough for skeletal growth, soft tissue growth and some left over to give the urine an adequate buffer value.

5. There must be sufficient chloride in the diet to satisfy the demands of volume regulation. Otherwise excess bicarbonate is generated to accompany sodium reabsorption causing alkalosis.

6. The diet should be designed with the objective of minimizing $[NA]_u$.

7. There is so little data in the literature that precise quantitative recommendations cannot be made. It is essential therefore that if the effect of a given diet on the whole body NB balance is to be known, metabolic balance studies must be performed.

Acknowledgement

Our particular thanks are due to Professor P. Kildeburg who with great patience took endless trouble to read and correct this chapter.

REFERENCES

1. Shohl A.T. & Sato A. (1924). Acid-base metabolism. I. Determination of base balance. *J. Biol. Chem.* **58**, 235–55.
2. Relman A.S., Lennon E.J., Lemann J., Jr & Connors H.P. (1961). Endogenous production of fixed acid and the measurement of the net balance of acid in normal subjects. *J. Clin. Invest.* **40**, 1621–30.
3. Lemann J., Jr, Lennon E.J., Goodman A.D., Litzow J.R. & Relman A.S. (1965). The balance of net acid in subjects given large loads of acid or alkali. *J. Clin. Invest.* **44**, 507–17.
4. Goodman A.D., Lemann J., Jr, Lennon E.J. & Relman A.S. (1965). Production, excretion and net balance of fixed acid in patients with renal acidosis. *J. Clin. Invest.* **44**, 495–506.
5. Lennon E.J., Lemann J., Jr & Litzow J.R. (1966). The effects of diet and stool composition on the net external acid balance of normal subjects. *J. Clin. Invest.* **45**, 1601–7.
6. Lemann J., Jr, Litzow J.R. & Lennon E.J. (1966). The effect of chronic acid loads in normal man: Further evidence for the participation of bone mineral in the defense against chronic metabolic acidosis. *J. Clin. Invest.* **45**, 1608–14.
7. Kildeberg P. (1981). *Quantitative Acid-Base Physiology. System Physiology and Pathophysiology of Renal, Gastrointestinal, and Skeletal Acid-Base Metabolism.* University Press, Odense, Denmark.
8. Kildeberg P. & Winters R.W. (1978). Balance of Net Acid: Concept, Measurement and Applications. *Adv. Pediatr.* **25**, 349–81.
9. Kildeberg P., Engel K. & Winters R.W. (1969). Balance of net acid in growing infants. Endogenous and transintestinal aspects. *Acta Paediatr. Scand* **58**, 321–9.
10. Slater J.E. (1961). Retention of nitrogen and minerals by babies 1 week old. *Br. J. Nutr.* **15**, 83–7.
11. Wamberg P., Kildeberg P. & Engel K. (1976). Balance of Net Base in the Rat. II. Reference Values in Relation to Growth Rate. *Biol. Noenat.* **28**, 171–90.

12. Pitts R.F. (1968). *Physiology of the Kidney and Body Fluids*. Year Book Medical Publishers Inc, Chicago.
13. Svenningson N.W. (1974). Renal acid base titration studies in infants with and without metabolic acidosis in the post neonatal period. *Pediat. Res.* **8**, 659–72.
14. Sulyok E. & Heim T. (1971). Assessment of maximal urinary acidification in premature infants. *Biol. Neonat.* **19**, 200–10.
15. Kildeberg P. (1964). Disturbances of hydrogen ion balance occuring in premature infants. II. Late Metabolic Acidosis. *Acta Paediatr. (Upsala)* **53**, 517–19.
16. Ranlov P. & Sigaard-Anderson O. (1965). Late metabolic acidosis in premature infants: Prevalence and significance. *Acta Paediatr.* (Upsala) **54**, 531–40.
17. Svenningsen N.W. & Lindquist B. (1973). Incidence of metabolic acidosis in term, preterm and small for gestational age infants in relation to dietary protein intake. *Acta Paediatr. Scand.* **62**, 1–10.
18. Raiha N.C.R., Heinonen K., Rassin D.K. & Gaull G.E. (1976). Milk protein quality and quantity in low birth weight infants: I. Metabolic responses and effects on growth. *Pediatrics* **62**, 659–74.
19. Laurenti F., Orzalezi M., Spennata G. & Marzetti G. (1971). Influenza della somministrazione di alcalinizzanti sull'accrescimento ponderale del prematuro con acidosi metabolica tardiva. *Min. Pediatr.* **23**, 267–77.
20. Schwartz G.J., Haycock G.B., Edelmann C.M., Jr & Spitzer A. (1978). Late metabolic acidosis: A reassessment of the definition. *J. Pediat.* **95** 102–7.
21. Senterre J. (1976). L'alimentation optimale du Premature. Thesis, University of Liege, Vaillant-Carmanne s.a., Liege.
22. Senterre J. & Lambrechts A. (1972). Nitrogen, fat and minerals balances in premature infants fed acidified or non-acidified half skimmed cow milk. *Biol. Neonat.* **20**, 107–119.
23. Glick H. & Allen A.C. (1971). Diet induced metabolic acidosis in prematurely born infants. *J. Pediatr.* **78**, 1061–2.
24. Healy C.E. (1972). Acidosis and failure to thrive in infants fed Nutramigen. *Pediatrics* **49**, 910.
25. Kildeberg P. & Winters R.W. (1972). Infant feeding and blood acid base status. *Pediatrics* **49**, 801–2.
26. Ashes R.S., Wisotsky D.H., Migel P.F., Seigle R.L. & Levy J. The dietary chloride deficiency syndrome occurring in a breast fed infant. *J. Pediatr.* **100**, 923–4.
27. Roy A., III & Arant B.S. (1979). Alkalosis from chloride deficient Neo-Mul-Soy. *N. Eng. J. Med.* **301**, 615.
28. Grossman H., Duggan E., McCamman S., Welchert E. & Gellerstein S. (1980). Dietary chloride deficiency syndrome. *Paediatrics* **66**, 366–74.

Feeding the Preterm Infant

15
Feeding: Methods
and Psychological Considerations

NUTRITIONAL BACKGROUND

It may be hard to achieve adequate nutrition in the very low birth weight (VLBW) infant during initial enteral feeding because of the immaturity of the gastrointestinal tract. The difficulty in achieving adequate nasogastric alimentation during the first days of life has led to a search for other ways of feeding, for example, total or partial parenteral nutrition or transpyloric feeding.

It is not within the scope of this book to discuss intravenous alimentation but, as the VLBW infant has high insensible water losses and impaired glucose homeostasis, with increased risk of dehydration and hypoglycaemia, fluid and nutrient requirements are usually provided from birth to some extent by the intravenous route. As total parenteral nutrition has not been proved to be safer than enteral feeding (1) and can lead to serious complications (2), enteral feeding must be started as soon as possible. Supplementary intravenous feeding allows the early provision of the necessary minimum nutrient intake with minimum initial weight loss (3), and until such time as oral feeding can be considered safe in a VLBW preterm infant, enteral intake must be given through a feeding tube leading into the gastrointestinal tract.

TUBE FEEDING

Tube fixation

Nasal tubes are easier to stabilize than oral ones, but occlusion of part of the nasal airway has been shown to interfere with respiration in the very tiny preterm infant (4,5). On the other hand, the better developed gag reflex in larger infants increases the possibility of displacement of oral tubes unless they are properly secured, for instance by the use of palatal plates (6,7).

Gastric feeding: intermittent gavage or continuous infusion

Intermittent gavage through an intragastric tube is simple and remains the usual practice for enteral feeding. It offers the possibility of an easily checked gastric residue before each meal and therefore an assessment of the gastric emptying capacity. Gastric emptying time is shorter with human milk than with formula (8), and may be decreased by prone or lateral position (9).

However, it increases with increasing energy density of formula (10), and the characteristics of the upper gastrointestinal tract of the preterm infant are such that difficulties with adequate enteral nutrition are common (11), especially when dealing with sick or very small infants. Inadequate gastric emptying (8,10,12), relatively incompetent lower oesophageal sphincter mechanism (13), and small stomach capacity all favour gastroesophageal reflux (14), regurgitation, and the risk of aspiration and apnoea (15). Furthermore, gastric distension may interfere with respiratory function (16–19). For all these reasons feeds may need to be given more frequently than in the full term infant and sometimes as often as hourly in order to reduce the feed volume. Hourly or two hourly feeding schedules require a lot of nursing time (20) and continuous gastric feed infusion may be considered as an alternative if careful attention is paid to the gastric residue (21,22).

When using the gastric route, either by continuous or bolus infusion, the stomach is still used as a reservoir with some digestive and functional activities. However, continuous infusion may have some possibly adverse metabolic effects. For example, in animals, differences in body composition (23,24,25) and organ size (26) have been reported according to whether feeding was intermittent or continuous. Metabolic and endocrine events seen in term babies fed intermittently were not seen in preterm infants given small meal volumes in a continuous or hourly schedule (27). Thus intermittent feeding may be important in the induction of metabolic and endocrine changes which occur in early postnatal life.

During continuous infusion of breast milk, nutrients (especially fat) may be lost within the syringes or the connecting tubing (28–31) which results in loss of energy. Such losses are less likely to occur with formulas, which are usually more stable than human milk. However, specially adapted preterm formulas with high energy and mineral content may clot within the feeding tubes (32).

Transpyloric feeding

Although continuous infusion minimizes the problems of gastric feeding, it does not abolish them. Rhea (33,34) and several subsequent authors have reported success with the use of transpyloric feeding (35–38), especially in the smallest and sickest infants in comparison with gastric feeding (35,39). The advantages claimed are minimal gastric distension, lower risk of aspiration and, at least during the first ten days of life, potentially greater volume tolerance with less initial weight loss than with nasogastric feeding. Three prospective controlled studies have compared transpyloric feeding with nasogastric intermittent gavage feeding (36,40,41): two found that transpyloric feeding allowed a larger volume intake to be tolerated and decreased the initial weight loss (36,41), although this advantage disappeared in most infants after the first two weeks of life. The third study did not find any advantage with transpyloric feeding (40). In one study (41) transpyloric feeding was found to be unsuccessful when respiratory assistance by mask was necessary, but no increase in complications was described when other types of ventilation were used (36,40). Two prospective studies compare continuous nasogastric and transpyloric feeding (37,42) but only one of them (37) concluded that there was an advantage in transpyloric feeding during the first two or three weeks of life.

Techniques of transpyloric intubation and their advantages and disadvantages have been recently reviewed (43,44).

Polyvinyl chloride tubes (PVC), which are easily positioned, have been found to harden (45,46) when left for several days in the duodenum, and perforations have been reported (45,47–49). Silastic tubes greatly reduce but do not abolish this complication (48), and are now commonly used, although they are more difficult to position because of their greater flexibility. Indeed the tip of the tube can double back into the stomach (leading to all the complications of gastric feeding) and even into the oesophagus, or may advance too far into the jejunum, causing malabsorption and diarrhoea.

In preterm infants transpyloric feeding is given continuously. This spreads the osmotic load of the feed which must be checked carefully as it may contribute to diarrhoea or NEC (50). There are no data on intermittent feeding via this route.

By-passing the stomach may have disadvantages from a nutritional point of view. Digestion of fat starts in the stomach (51,52,53) and jejunal placement of a feeding tube is associated with fat malabsorption (54). This may be minimized by duodenal placement (37).

Qualitative changes in the upper gastrointestinal microflora (with higher *E. Coli* counts) have been described during transpyloric feeding (55), and continuous drip feeds are more prone to contamination (56). Therefore, great attention must be paid to handling techniques and to the initial bacteriological content of milk given.

Other complications related to transpyloric feeding include diarrhoea and bilious vomiting which are usually minor and may be controlled by reducing the volume or checking the position of the tube. Pyloric stenosis has been described with prolonged nasojejunal feeding (57,58). Necrotizing enterocolitis (NEC) causes more concern (59), although data on the incidence of NEC during transpyloric feeding are controversial. In controlled studies (36,37,40,41) NEC has not been proven to be more frequent during transpyloric than during nasogastric feeding.

SUCKING

LBW infants are often unable to suck and swallow properly. However, their ability to deal with these functions is often under-estimated. Successful breast and/or bottle feeding can be achieved in infants with a mean body weight of 1300 grams and a mean postnatal age of 11 days (60). Therefore, the sucking ability of preterm infants, including those below 1500 grams, should be frequently tested, bearing in mind that oral feeding may result in an impairment of ventilation (19) and in apnoea (61).

When an infant is tube fed either by intermittent gavage or continuously, there is evidence (62,63) of a beneficial effect in allowing the baby to suck intermittently from a nipple. This so-called 'non-nutritive sucking' has been claimed to accelerate the maturation of the sucking reflex, thus permitting an earlier introduction of bottle or breast feeding. Faster weight gain has also been reported, resulting in earlier discharge from hospital. Whether this latter finding results from a decreased level of activity (64), or from a better nutrient absorption due to increased lingual lipase secretion, or both, is not clear.

SOME PSYCHOLOGICAL CONSIDERATIONS

It was not our remit to consider general aspects of the care of the preterm baby. Nevertheless where necessary we have touched on those aspects of general care which clearly overlap with the baby's nutrition (e.g. thermoregulation in Chapter 3). In the same way, the psychological aspects of feeding are mentioned briefly. In recent years the importance of these aspects of neonatal care has been rediscovered. There are a number of reviews concerning early mother and child interaction (65–66) including the role of feeding in its development (67).

It is well known that the woman's reactions to preterm delivery follow a predictable sequence of emotional events: from a mourning phase for the anticipatory loss of her baby, through a phase of guilt and depression for not having been able to deliver a normal term infant, to the gradual resumption of the relational process with her infant and the recognition of the special needs of her premature baby.

This normal sequence of emotional events can be easily upset or distorted, leading to a variety of disturbances of mothering behaviour and of child development, including some well defined clinical entities, such as a failure to thrive without an organic cause or a battered child syndrome, which have been shown to be significantly more frequent in LBW infants.

Early and prolonged separation between mother and infant is an important risk factor for the derangement of the normal process of maternal attachment and bonding. It is likely that this could happen not only because of physical separation, but also when strong psychological and emotional barriers are present. The mother of a premature infant, or of a sick baby in general, often feels that the child 'belongs' to the hospital and this sensation of being excluded from the care of her baby is very frustrating to her and enhances the feeling that there is something very wrong with the baby. Feeding is a 'normal' process and carries with it a connotation of 'normality' for the baby which is being fed. Knowing that the baby is fed with her milk or being involved in any way with the feeding routine of her infant is therefore reassuring for the mother.

Nursery routines should thus be geared toward encouraging the mother to play an active role in feeding her baby, and any occasion for the mother to touch, caress or fondle her baby should be facilitated. She should be able to look in his eyes and speak to him, since this is important for an optimal interaction between mother and baby.

Furthermore, the simultaneous presence of many parents in the Unit at feeding time enhances a more sociable and less medicalized atmosphere, where parents interact among themselves deriving reciprocal support in dealing with the problems of their respective infants.

The main concept is that feeding the baby is a crucial part of a complex relational system which includes the baby, the mother and father, the siblings, the medical and paramedical personnel and all the other people present in the nursery. The goal is not only to discharge a well nourished infant, but also one who is happy, with a happy mother and with an optimal relationship with his parents.

Paediatricians concerned with the nutritional well being of the child are necessarily involved with his psychological well being at the same time.

GUIDELINES

Enteral feeding should be introduced as soon as it is safe to do so.

1 Intermittent gastric tube feeding seems more physiological than transpyloric feeding and whenever possible should be preferred.
2 When there are feeding difficulties such as regurgitation, poor gastric

emptying or gastric distension, continuous gastric feeding or even transpyloric feeding may be necessary, as they are useful alternatives either to reduced oral feeding or to total parenteral nutrition.

3 The success of any feeding technique is at least partly the result of the skill of the staff of the Unit in following their own practised routines.

4 Nursery routines should encourage the mother to play an active role in feeding. This will help her to become confident in the care of her baby.

REFERENCES

1. Glass E.J., Hume R., Lang M.A. & Forfar J.O. (1984). Parenteral nutrition compared with transpyloric feeding. *Arch. Dis. Child.* **59**, 131–5.
2. Bryan M.H., Wei P., Hamilton J.R., Chance G.W. & Swyer P.R. (1973). Supplemental intravenous alimentation in low-birth-weight infants. *J. Pediatr.* **82**, 940–4.
3. Brans Y.W. (1977). Parenteral nutrition of the very low birth weight neonate: a critical view. *Clin. Perinatol.* **44**, 367–76.
4. Stocks J. (1980). Effects of nasogastric tubes on nasal resistance during infancy. *Arch. Dis. Child.* **55**, 17–21.
5. Someren V.V., Linnett S.J., Stothers J.K. & Sullivan P.G. (1984). An investigation into the benefits of resiting nasoenteric feeding tubes. *Pediatrics* **74**, 379–83.
6. Sullivan P.G. (1982). An appliance to support oral intubation in the premature. *Br. Dent. J.* **152**, 191–5.
7. Errenberg A. & Nowak A.J. (1984). Appliance for stabilizing orogastric and orotracheal tubes in infants. *Crit. Care Med.* **12**, 669–71.
8. Cavell B. (1979). Gastric emptying in preterm infants. *Acta Paediatr. Scand.* **68**, 725—30.
9. Yu V.Y.H. (1975). Effect of body position on gastric emptying in the neonate. *Arch. Dis. Child.* **50**, 500–4.
10. Siegel M., Lebenthal E. & Krantz B. (1984). Effect of caloric density on gastric emptying in premature infants. *J. Pediatr.* **104**, 118—22.
11. Siegel M. & Lebenthal E. (1981). Developmental of gastrointestinal motility and gastric emptying during the fetal newborn periods. In: *Textbook of Gastroenterology and Nutrition in Infancy*, (ed. E. Lebenthal) pp. 121–38. Raven Press, New York.
12. Gupta M. & Brans Y.W. (1978). Gastric retention in neonates. *Pediatrics* **62**, 26–9.
13. Biox-Ochoa J. & Canals J. (1976). Maturation of the lower esophagus. *J. Pediatr. Surg.* **11**, 749–56.
14. Hillemeier A.C., Lange R., McCallum R., Seashore J. & Gryboski J. (1981). Delayed gastric emptying in infants with gastroesophageal reflux. *J. Pediatr.* **98**, 190–3.
15. Herbst J.J., Minton S.D. & Book L.S. (1979). Gastroesophageal reflux causing respiratory distress and apnea in newborn infants. *J. Pediatr.* **95**, 763–8.
16. Pitcher-Wilmott R., Shutack J.G. & Fow W.W. (1979). Decreased lung volume after nasogastric feeding of neonates recovering from respiratory distress. *J. Pediatr.* **95**, 119–21.
17. Herrell N., Martin R.J. & Faranoff A. (1980). Arterial oxygen tension during nasogastric feeding in the preterm infant. *J. Pediatr.* **96**, 914–16.
18. Yu V.Y.H. (1976). Cardiorespiratory response to feeding in newborn infants. *Arch. Dis. Child.* **51**, 305–9.
19. Shirpuri C.R., Martin R.S., Carlo W.A. & Faranoff A.M. (1983). Decreased ventilation in preterm infants during oral feeding. *J. Pediatr.* **103**, 285–9.
20. Whitfield M.F. (1981). Transpyloric feeding in infants undergoing intensive care. *Arch. Dis. Child.* **56**, 571–2.
21. Landwith J. (1972). Continuous nasogastric infusion versus total intravenous alimentation. *J. Pediatr.* **81**, 1037–8.

22. Valman H.B., Heath C.D. & Brown R.J.K. (1972). Continuous intragastric milk feeding in infants of low birth weight. *Br. Med. J.* 3, 547–50.
23. Ozelci A., Romso D.R. & Leveille G.A. (1977). Influence of diet composition on nitrogen balance and body composition in meal eating and nibling rats. *J. Nutr.* 107, 1768–74.
24. Anderson T.A., Raffety C.J., Birkhofer K.K. & Fomon S.J. (1980). Effect of feeding frequency on growth and body composition of gastrotomized rat pups. *J. Nutr.* 110, 2374–80.
25. Heggeness F.N. (1965). Effect of intermittent food restriction on growth, food utilization and body composition on rat. *J. Nutr.* 86, 265–70.
26. Pockenee R.C. & Heaton F.N. (1976). The effect of feeding frequency on the growth and composition of individual organs in the rat. *Br. J. Nutr.* 35, 97–104.
27. Lucas A., Bloom S.R. & Aynsley Green A. (1978). Metabolic and endocrine events at the time of the first feed of human milk in preterm and term infants. *Arch. Dis. Child.* 53, 731–6.
28. Greer F.R., McCormick A. & Locker J. (1984). Changes in fat concentration of human milk during delivery by intermittent bolus and continuous mechanical pump infusion. *J. Pediatr.* 105, 745–9.
29. Brooke O.G. & Barley J. (1978). Loss of energy during continuous infusion of breast milk. *Arch. Dis. Child.* 53, 344–5.
30. Narayanan I., Singh B. & Harvey D. (1984). Fat loss during feeding of human milk. *Arch Dis. Child.* 59, 475–7.
31. Stocks R.J., Davies D.P., Allen F. & Sewell D. (1985). Loss of breast milk nutrients during tube feeding. *Arch. Dis. Child.* 60, 164–6.
32. Moyer L. & Chan G.M. (1982). Clotted feeding tubes with transpyloric feeding of premature infant formula. *J. Pediatr. Gastr. Nutr.* 1, 55—7.
33. Rhea J.W., Ghazzawi O. & Weidman W. (1973). Nasojejunal feeding: an improved device and intubation technique. *J. Pediatr.* 82, 951–4.
34. Rhea J.W., Ahmad M.S. & Mange M.S. (1975). Nasojejunal (transpyloric) feeding: a commentary. *J. Pediatr.* 96, 451–2.
35. Minoli I., Moro G. & Ovadia M.F. (1978). Nasoduodenal feeding in high risk newborns. *Acta Paediatr. Scand.* 67, 161–8.
36. Wells D.H. & Dackman R.D. (1975). Nasojejunal feeding in LBW infants. *J. Pediatr.* 87, 276–9.
37. Van Caillie M. & Powell G.K. (1975). Nasoduodenal versus nasogastric feeding in the very low birth weight infant. *Pediatrics* 56, 1065–72.
38. Meunier G., Putet G. & Salle B. (1982). Alimentation entérale continue par sonde nasoduodénale chez le prématuré de poids de naissance <1200 g. *Arch. Fr. Pediatr.* 39, 79–83.
39. Cheek J.A. & Staub G.F. (1973). Nasojejunal alimentation for premature and full term newborn infants. *J. Pediatr.* 82, 955–62.
40. Pereira G.R. & Lemons J.A. (1981). Controlled study of transpyloric and intermittent gavage feeding in the small preterm infant. *Pediatrics* 67, 68–72.
41. Beddis I. & McKenzie S. (1979). Transpyloric feeding in the very low birth weight (1500 g and below) infant. *Arch. Dis. Child.* 54, 213–17.
42. Whitfield M.F. (1982). Poor weight gain of the low birth weight infant fed nasojejunally. *Arch. Dis. Child.* 57, 597–601.
43. Topper W.H. (1981). Enteral feeding methods for compromised neonates and infants. In: *Textbook of Gastroenterology and Nutrition in Infancy*, Vol. 1, (ed. E. Lebenthal) pp. 647–58. Raven Press, New York.
44. Dryburgh E. (1982). Transpyloric feeding. In: *Topics in Perinatal Medicine II* (ed. B.A. Wharton) 75—86. Pitman, London.
45. Boros S. & Reynolds J.W. (1974). Duodenal perforation, a complication of neonatal nasojejunal feeding. *J. Pediatr.* 85, 107–8.
46. Hayhurst E.G. & Wyman M. (1975). Morbidity associated with prolonged use of polyvinyl feeding tubes. *Am. J. Dis. Child.* 129, 72–4.

47. Fogle R.S., Smith W.L. & Gresham E.L. (1978). Perforation of feeding tube into right pelvis. *J. Pediatr.* **93**, 122–4.
48. Rodriguez J.P., Guero J., Frias E.G. & Omenaca F. (1978). Duodenorenal perforation in a neonate by a tube of silicone rubber during traspyloric feeding. *J. Pediatr.* **92**, 113–16.
49. Chen W.J. & Wong P.W.K. (1974). Intestinal complication of nasojejunal feeding in low birth weight infants. *J. Pediatr.* **85**, 109–10.
50. Book L.S., Herbst J.J., Atherton S.O. & Jung A.L. (1975). Necrotising enterocolitis in low birth weight infants fed an elemental formula. *J. Pediatr.* **87**, 602–9.
51. Hamosh M. (1981). Oral lipases and lipid digestion during the neonatal period. In: *Textbook of Gastroenterology and Nutrition in Infancy.* Vol. 1, (ed. E. Lebenthal), pp. 445–63. Raven Press, New York.
52. Liao T.H., Hamosh P. & Hamosh M. (1984). Fat digestion by lingual lipase: mechanism of lipolysis in the stomach and upper small intestine. *Pediatr. Res.* **18**, 402–9.
53. Fink C.S. & Hamosh M. (1984). Fat digestion in the stomach: stability of lingual lipase in the gastric environment. *Pediatr. Res.* **18**, 248–54.
54. Roy R.N., Pollnitz R.P., Hamilton J.R. & Chance G.W. (1977). Impaired assimilation of nasojejunal feeds in healthy low birth weight newborn infants. *J. Pediatr.* **90**, 431–4.
55. Challacombe D. (1974). Bacterial microflora in infants receiving nasojejunal tube feeding. *J. Pediatr.* **85**, 113.
56. Schreiner R.L., Eitzen H., Gfell M.A., Kress S., Gresham E.L., French M. & Moye L. (1979). Environmental contamination of continuous drip feedings. *Pediatrics* **63**, 232–7.
57. Raine P.A.M., Goel K.M., Young D.G., Galea P., McLaurin J.C., Ford J. & Sweetem A. (1982). Pyloric stenosis and transpyloric feeding. *Lancet* **ii**, 821–2.
58. Evans N.J. (1982). Pyloric stenosis in premature infants after transpyloric feeding. *Lancet* **ii**, 665.
59. Vasquez C., Arroyos A., Val I. & Sole A. (1980). Necrotising enterocolitis. Increased incidence in infant receiving nasoduodenal feeding. *Arch. Dis. Child.* **55**, 826.
60. Pearce J.L. & Buchanan L.F. (1980). Breast milk and breast feeding in very low birth weight infants. *Arch. Dis. Child.* **54**, 897–9.
61. Guilleminault G. & Coons S. (1984). Apnea and bradycardia during feeding in infants weighing [< 2000 g. *J. Pediatr.* **104**, 932–5.
62. Field T., Ignatoff E., Stringer S., Brennan J., Greenberg R., Widmayer S. & Anderson G.C. (1982). Non nutritive sucking during tube feedings: effects on preterm neonates in an intensive care unit. *Pediatrics* **70**, 381–4.
63. Bernbaum J.C., Pereira G.R., Watkins J.B. & Peckham J. (1983). Non nutritive sucking during gavage feeding enhances growth and maturation in premature infants. *Pediatrics* **71**, 41–5.
64. Field T. & Golbdson E. (1984). Pacifying effects of non nutritive sucking on term and preterm neonates during heelstick procedures. *Pediatrics* **74**, 1012–15.
65. Klaus M.H. & Kennel J.H. (1982). *Parent—Infant Bonding.* Mosby, St Louis.
66. Taylor P.M., ed. (1980). *Parent—Infant Relationships.* Green and Stratton, New York.
67. Taylor P.M., Taylor F.H., Maloni J.A., Campbell S.B. & Cannon M. (1985). Effects of extra early mother–infant contact. *Acta Paediatr. Scand.* (Suppl.) **319**. Passim.
68. Richards M.P.M. (1982). Breast feeding and the mother infant relationship. *Acta Paediatr. Scand.* (Suppl.) **299**, 33–7.

16

The Use of Breast Milk

Human milk is a complex and unique fluid containing nutritional compounds for the developing infant but also a large variety of soluble and insoluble components exhibiting important non-nutritional properties.

The chemical composition of human milk shows considerable variation between different individuals and in the same individual at different times of lactation (1), as well as between samples obtained from mothers of LBW infants and term infants (2,3). These differences in the nutrient composition may reflect differences in nutritive requirements of infants at different stages of maturity and physiological as well as biochemical development.

The nutritional components in human milk have been discussed in the various chapters on specific nutrients.

NON-NUTRITIONAL COMPONENTS IN HUMAN MILK

Host resistance factors

There is clear evidence that breast-fed infants are better protected for gastrointestinal as well as respiratory infections (4,5). Fresh human milk contains a wealth of components that provide specific as well as non-specific defences against infectious agents and other macromolecules.

These components include immunocompetent T and B lymphocytes, polymorphonuclear leucocytes (6–8), immunoglobulins, especially secretory IgA (9,10) and components of the complement system (11).

Human milk also contains specific binding proteins which bind nutrients needed for the growth of bacteria. Lactoferrin is an iron binding protein. Binding proteins for folic acid and vitamin B_{12} are also found (12). Additional specific soluble factors against streptococci, staphylococci and viruses have been identified (13,14).

An interesting recent development is the observation that human milk has a high content of complex carboydrates. Of these the oligosaccharides are of major interest. The structure of some of the milk oligosaccharides are similar

201

or identical to cell surface carbohydrates. A possible physiological role for milk oligosaccharides could be that they act as free receptors and thereby prevent bacterial adhesion to the cell surfaces (15).

Enzymes and hormones

There are at least 60 enzymes in human milk (16) but very little is known about their *in vivo* function and importance for the developing human neonate. Some enzymes in human milk may be present as a result of 'leakage' from the mammary gland tissue and play little or no physiological role, others have important functions. One enzyme which has been much studied and has an important physiological function is the bile salt stimulated lipase (17). This lipase is only found in the milk of primates. Newborn infants and especially preterm infants have a low pancreatic lipase activity and a low intraluminal bile salt concentration as well as a low pool size (18,19). These factors explain the incomplete lipid absorption in the preterm infant. If the bile salt stimulated lipase is destroyed in the milk by heating the fat absorption from human milk may be as low as 50% and less (20). From fresh human milk the fat absorption is over 90%, this would suggest that bile salt stimulated lipase has a very important function for the lipid absorption in the preterm infant (21).

Amylase is another enzyme in human milk which may have an important function during the neonatal period when both salivary and pancreatic amylase activity is low (22).

Human milk has also been found to contain protease inhibitors such as α_1-antitrypsin and α_1-antichymotrypsin (23). Whether the protease inhibitors have a physiological function in the gastrointestinal tract of the infant is not known with certainty. Sulphydryl oxidases are a class of enzymes originally found in bovine milk which catalyse the synthesis of disulphide bonds. Sulphydryl oxidase is present in human milk and is very stable in an acid environment. Human milk sulphydryl oxidase is also resistant to gut proteases (24). The *in vivo* function of sulphydryl oxidases in the gastrointestinal tract of the infant needs further elucidation.

Several hormones have been detected in human milk (25). However, it remains to be studied whether hormones present in milk are of physiological significance to the newborn infant. It has been suggested that breast feeding prevents the symptoms of neonatal hypothyroidism due to the availability of thyroid hormones in human milk (26).

Growth factors

These are substances that can be shown to modify the growth and proliferation of cells. Their physiological function in the neonate are not well defined.

Taurine, a sulphur containing amino acid which is present in the non-protein nitrogen fraction of human milk has recently been shown to have a strong proliferative effect on cultured human lymphoblastoid cells (27). The possible importance of taurine for the proliferation and development of the gastrointestinal tract needs further critical investigation. However, it should be emphasized, from the point of view of feeding the very low birthweight (VLBW) infant, that most presently available formulas contain very little taurine although some formulas are taurine supplemented.

Recent studies have demonstrated that human milk contains several proteins that promote growth in cultured cells. The best defined is epidermal growth factor EGF (28) and nerve growth factor NFG. EGF is the most potent stimulator of epidermal and epithelial tissue growth and differentiation, whereas NGF is essential for the development of sympathetic and sensory neurons. In adult mice EGF and NGF are present in high concentration in the submaxillary gland and the saliva. Salivary EGF and NGF is passed into the gastrointestinal tract. In suckling mice these factors are absent from the salivary gland and saliva, but present in milk, and it is thus interesting to speculate that milk may provide these growth factors during the maturation of the salivary production.

DONOR BREAST MILK

Breast milk can be collected either by expressing milk by hand or by pump or by collecting 'drip milk' (29). A comparison of fat concentration of drip milk with expressed breast milk (29) shows that expressed milk is substantially higher in fat concentration and therefore the energy content than drip milk. The fat content of human milk varies widely from individual to individual (see chapter on fat) and therefore unless all individual donor milk samples can be measured for fat content it is wise to pool several milk samples so that fat content is more uniform.

Milk from mothers of premature infants, especially during the first two weeks after delivery contains more energy, higher concentration of fat, protein and sodium and lower concentrations of lactose, calcium and phosphorus than milk from mothers of term infants (30–33).

USE OF HUMAN MILK FOR FEEDING PRETERM INFANTS

The many non-nutritional components in fresh human milk provide important factors for the immature organism and human milk should preferentially be given to these infants at least for the first months after birth. Pooled human milk from mothers of term infants does not always meet all the nutritional requirements of VLBW infants (2). It would therefore be necessary to provide quality control for mature milk to ensure that major nutrients such as protein, fat, minerals are present in concentrations suitable for the needs of the premature infants who will get the milk. Supplementation may become necessary (see chapters on specific nutrients protein, sodium, calcium, phosphorus, and trace minerals). The higher fat and protein content of preterm milk may, however, be sufficient to meet the requirements for preterm infants when such milk is consumed at volumes of 180–200 ml/kg per day.

Recent research has developed methods to prepare fractions from human milk which can be stored and used for enrichment of donor milk in order to design 'human milk formula' which may fulfill the special nutritional needs of VLBW infants (34–36). Mixtures of whey-predominant protein, carbohydrate, calcium, phosphate, trace minerals and vitamins for addition to human milk intended for VLBW infants have also been developed by commercial formula manufacturers (37). Few or no published studies on the nutritional effects of fortified human milk have been reported.

EFFECTS OF HEAT TREATMENT ON HUMAN MILK COMPONENTS

Most proteins are denatured when exposed to heat and therefore it is evident that heating milk will have an adverse effect on many protein components which may have a physiologically important function in milk. The data found in the literature is mostly limited to describe the effects on the anti-infective protein fractions in human milk (38). Lysozyme and SIgA does not lose much activity at heating up to 62.5 but above this temperature activity is lost very rapidly (38). Other factors such as time of reaching a specific temperature, time of cooling and the volumes processed will also influence the results. Human milk enzymes are also very sensitive to heat. Bile salt stimulated lipase rapidly loses activity when incubated at 50°C and after 5 minutes 50% of the activity is lost (39). Holder pasteurization (62.5°C for 30 minutes) completely inactivates sulphydryl oxidases in human milk (24). Since several studies have demonstrated that bacteria multiplies much more rapidly when added to heat treated human milk than to raw milk (40), this should be taken into consideration if pasteurized milk is used for LBW infants.

GUIDELINES

1 The milk of the mother of a baby who is delivered preterm if fed at 180–200 ml/kg each day may provide adequate nutrition in many instances.

2 Banked human milk may also be used but there is usually a need to supplement this with sodium, phosphate, and perhaps protein and calcium (see previous chapters).

3 Vitamin supplements will be necessary and iron should be introduced from not later than 8 weeks of age (see previous chapters).

4 Despite the effects of heat treatment on various components it has been advised that whenever donor milk is used for premature infants it should be heat treated due to the possibility of virus infection (CMV, HTLV-III). This matter is still controversial.

REFERENCES

1. Lönnerdal B., Forsum E. & Hambraeus L. (1976). The protein content of human milk. I. A transversal study of Swedish normal mothers. *Nutr. rep. Int.* **13**, 125–34.
2. Hibberd C.M., Brooke O.G., Carter N.D., Hang M. & Harzer G. (1982). Variation in the composition of breast milk during the first 5 weeks of lactation: implications for the feeding of preterm infants. *Arch. Dis. Child.* **57**, 658–62.
3. Butte N.F., Garza C., Johnson C.A., O'Brian Smith E. & Nichols B.L. (1984). Longitudinal changes in milk composition of mothers delivering preterm and term infants. *Early Hum. Dev.* **9**, 153–62.
4. Mata L.J. & Wyatt R.G. (1971). The uniqueness of human milk. Host resistance to infection. *Am. J. Clin. Nutr.* **24**, 976.
5. Hanson L.A. & Winberg J. (1972). Breast milk and defense against infection in the newborn. *Arch. Dis. Child.* **47**, 845–8.
6. Welsh J.K. & May J.T. (1979). Anti-infective properties of breast milk. *J. Pediatr.* **94**, 1–9.
7. Faden H. & Ogra P.L. (1981). Breast milk as an immunologic vehicle for transport of immunocompetence. In: *Textbook of Gastroenterology and Nutrition in Infancy*, Vol. 1. (ed. E. Lebenthal) pp. 355–61. Raven Press, New York.
8. Pitt J. (1975). Passive transfer of milk phagocytesmechanisms of protection in necrotizing entero-colitis. In: *Necrotizing Enterocolitis in the Newborn Infant*. Sixty-eighth Ross Conference on Pediatric Research, 52.
9. Ogra P.L. & Dayton D.H., eds (1980). *Immunology of Breast Milk*. Raven Press, New York.
10. Goldblum R.M., Attlstedt S., Carlsson B. *et al.* (1978). Antibody forming cells in human cholostrum. *Nature* **257**, 797.
11. Chandra R.K. (1978). Immunological aspects of human milk. *Nutr. Rev.* **36**, 265.
12. Bullen J.J. (1976). Iron-binding proteins and other factors in milk responsible for resistance to Eschericha coli. In: *Acute Diarrhoea in Childhood*, CIBA Foundation Symposium 42. Elsevier (North Holland) Exerpta Medica, Amsterdam.
13. György P. (1967). Human milk and resistance to infection. In: *Nutrition and Infection*. Ciba Foundation Study Group 31. p.59. Little, Brown & Co., Boston.
14. Ogra P.L. & Greene H.L. (1982). Human milk and breast feeding: an update on the state of the art. *Pediatr. Res.* **16**, 266–71.

15. Lundblad A. (1984). Human milk oligosaccharides. Presented at the Nordic Research Seminar on Breast Milk Composition and Relation to Nutritional Status of the Mother. Öregrund, Sweden, February 1984.

16. Shahani K.M., Kwan A.J. & Friend B.A. (1980). Role and significance of enzymes in human milk. *Am. J. Clin. Nutr.* **33**, 1861–9.

17. Hernell O. & Olivecrona I. (1974). Human Milk lipases. II. Bile Salt-stimulated lipase. *Biochim. Biophys. Acta.* **369**, 234–8.

18. Järvenpää A.-L., Rassin D.K., Kuitunen P., Gaull G.E. & Räihä N.C.R. (1983). Feeding the low-birth-weight infant. III. Diet influences bile acid metabolism. *Pediatrics* **72**, 677–83.

19. Watkins J.B., Järvenpää A.-L., Szczepanik Van-Leeuwen P., Klein P.D., Rassin D.K., Gaull G. & Räihä N.C.R. (1983). Feeding the low-birth-weight infant: Effects of taurine, cholesterol and human milk on bile acid kinetics. *Gastroenterology* **85**, 793–800.

20. Voyer M., Nobre R., Antener I., Colin J., Charlas J. & Satgé P. (1979). Alimentation des prématurés avec un lait industriel contenant des triglycérides a chaine moyenne. *Ann. Pediatr.* **26**, 417–32.

21. Järvenpää A.-L. (1983). Feeding the low birth weight infant: IV. Fat absorption as a function of diet and duodenal bile acids. *Pediatrics* **72**, 684–9.

22. Lindberg T. & Skude G. (1982). Amylase in human milk. *Pediatrics* **70**, 235—8.

23. Lindberg T., Ohlsson K. & Weström B. (1982). Protease inhibitors and their relation to protease activity in human milk. *Pediatr. Res.* **16**, 479—83.

24. Gaull G.E., Isaacs L.E., Wright C.E., Krueger L. & Tallan H.H. (1984). Growth modulators in human milk: implications for milk banking. In: *Human Milk Banking* (eds A.F. Williams & J.D. Baum). Nestlé Nutrition Workshop, Vevey/Raven Press, New York.

25. Koldovsky O. (1980). Hormones in milk: are they an important component of the nutrition of the neonate? Seventy-Ninth Ross Conference on Pediatric Research, Ross Laboratories, Columbus, Ohio, USA. p. 62.

26. Bode H.H., Varjonack W.J., Crawford J.D. (1978). Mitigation of cretinism by breast-feeding. *Pediatrics* **62**, 13—16.

27. Wright C.E., Schweitzer L.B., Billam B.M., Tallan H.H. & Gaull G.E. (in press). Taurine augments growth of cultured human B lymphoblastoid cells. *Science* (in press).

28. Carpenter G. (1980). Epidermal growth factor is a major growth-promoting agent in human milk. *Science* **210**, 198—201.

29. Baum J.D. (1982). Donor breast milk. *Acta Paediatr. Scand.* (Suppl.) **299**, 51.

30. Atkinson S.A., Anderson G.H. & Bryan M.H. (1980). Human milk: Comparison of the nitrogen composition in milk from mothers of premature and full-term infants. *Am. J. Clin. Nutr.* **33**, 811–15.

31. Gross S.J., David R.J., Bauman L. *et al.* (1980). Nutritional composition of milk produced by mothers delivering preterm. *J. Pediatr.* **96**, 641–4.

32. Anderson G.H., Atkinson S.A. & Bryan M.H. (1981). Energy and macronutrient content of human milk during early lactation from mothers giving birth prematurely and at term. *Am. J. Clin. Nutr.* **34**, 258–65.

33. Lemons J.A., Boye L., Hall D. *et al.* (1982). Differences in the composition of preterm and term human milk during early lactation. *Pediatr. Res.* **16**, 113–17.

34. Lucas A., Lucas P., Chavin S.I., Lyster R.L.J. & Baum J.D. (1980). A human milk formula. *Early Hum. Dev.* **4/1**, 15–21.

35. Hagelberg S., Lindblad B.S., Lundsjö A., Carlsson B., Fonden R., Fujita H., Lassfolk G. & Lindqvist B. (1982). The protein tolerance of very low birth weight infants fed human milk protein enriched mother's milk. *Acta Paediatr. (Scand.)* **71**, 597—601.

36. Hylmö P., Polberger S., Axelsson I., Jakobsson I. & Räihä N. (1984). Preparation of fat and protein from banked human milk: its use in feeding very low birth weight infants. In: *Human Milk Banking*, (eds A.F. Williams & J.D. Baum) pp. 55–61. Nestlé Nutrition Workshop, Vevey/Raven Press, New York.

37. American Academy of Pediatrics, Committee on Nutrition (1985). Nutritional needs of low-birth-weight infants. *Pediatrics* 75, 976–85.

38. Björksten B., Burman L.G., de Chateau P., Fredrikzon B., Gothefors L. & Hernell O. (1980). Collecting and banking human milk: to heat or not to heat? *Br. Med. J.* 281, 765.

39. Hernell O. (1975). Human Milk lipases. III. Physiological implications of the bile salt stimulated lipase. *Eur. J. Clin. Invest.* 5, 267—72.

40. Aernandez J., Lemons P., Lemons J. & Todd J. (1979). Effect of storage process on the bacterial growth-inhibiting activity of human breast milk. *Pediatrics* 63, 597—601.

17

The Use of Formulas

If the decision is made to feed the baby a formula, how much should be given, what should it contain, how should it be manufactured, how should it be presented, and what information should be available?

VOLUME OF INTAKE OF A FORMULA, ENERGY DENSITY OF THE FORMULA, AND ENERGY INTAKE BY THE BABY

The guideline for energy intake (see Energy, Chapter 3) is 110–165 kcal/kg and for energy density is 65–85 kcal/kg. Therefore, the range of fluid intake to *provide recommended energy intake* is 130–200 ml/kg, although in normal circumstances the intake will not be below 150. Intakes of water above and below this range may be required (see Water, Chapter 2), but when this occurs it should be seen as the priority of water balance over-riding the requirements of other nutrients.

Figure 17.1 shows the relationship of these three measurements. Not all combinations of energy density and energy intake are possible, e.g. if the energy density of the formula used is 65 kcal per 100 ml then an energy intake greater than 130 kcal kg cannot be achieved since the volume required would exceed the upper guidelines of 200 ml/kg.

In most enteral feeding regimens volumes commence at 40–60 ml/kg per day, and increase in daily increments of 20–30 ml/kg per day. Light for gestational age babies commonly receive volumes in the upper limits of this range to achieve an adequate energy intake and so avoid hypoglycaemia.

NUTRIENT COMPOSITION OF A FORMULA

Table 17.1 at the end of this chapter shows the guideline range for nutrients in a formula. In general the definitive guidelines presented in the earlier chapters (3–15) have been expressed per unit energy (i.e. per 100 kcal), e.g. protein, fat, calcium, etc., but for certain nutrients where their handling is closely related to water the guidelines have been expressed per unit volume (i.e. per 100 ml), e.g. electrolytes, and in some instances in other terms as well (e.g. vitamins E and B6).

A single guideline cannot be considered in isolation and we have examined how the various limitations interrelate. This has usually involved an amount of simple but tedious mathematics so that a nutrient limit expressed in grams per 100 kcal is also converted to nutrient per 100 ml of formula and nutrient per kg of body weight. However, some mathematical conversions from one guideline result in a figure which is not in keeping with another guideline and so the simple mathematical conversion does not appear in the table. Some of these points are illustrated, in further detail, in the examples below.

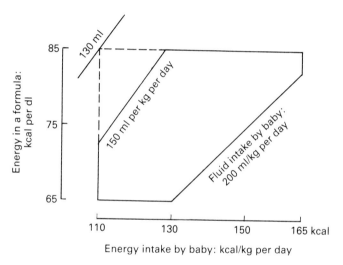

Fig. 17.1. Relationships between volume of intake, energy density of a formula, and energy intake by the baby.

Protein and energy (Fig. 17.2)

The figure is in two parts. In the upper part of the figure the six sided box indicates the limits implied by the recommendations for protein and energy, i.e. on the y axis: a protein energy ratio of 2.25 to 3.1 g per 100 kcal/kg per day. In addition, the sloping, slightly curved, lines show the intake of protein per kg body weight of the baby allowed by the guidelines, i.e. 2.9–4.0 g/kg per day. Therefore, points within the box are allowed by the guidelines but points outside the box are not.

The lower part of the figure indicates how a particular energy intake can be achieved by a baby within the recommendations, i.e. on the y axis: consuming a formula providing 65–85 kcal/dl; on the x axis a fluid intake of 130–200 ml/kg per day.

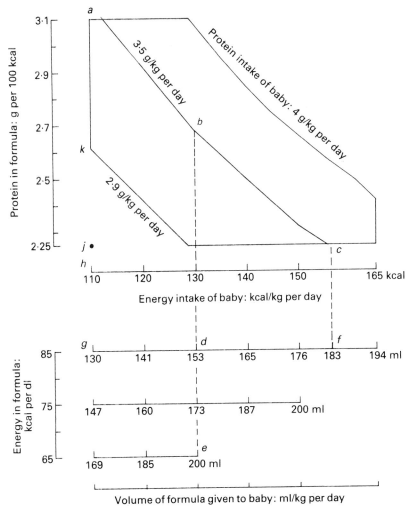

Fig. 17.2. Recommendations concerning protein: expressed g per 100 kcal for the recommended range of energy intake; also observing the recommended maximum and minimum intakes by the baby when expressed as g per kg body weight.

Example 1

Suppose the aim is to provide a protein intake of 3.5 g/kg within the permitted guidelines:

1   Looking at the box a protein intake of 3.5 g/kg is indicated by the line a b c; the intake could be achieved by feeding a formula containing 2.7 g per 100 kcal at 130 kcal/kg per day (point b). From this point move down to the lower box along line b d e. An energy intake of 130 kcal/kg could be achieved by feeding a

formula between the limits of 85 kcal/dl at 153 ml/kg (point d) and 65 kcal/dl at 200 ml/kg (point e).

2   Suppose instead that the intake of 3.5 g/kg were achieved by feeding a formula containing 2.25 g of protein at 156 kcal/kg per day (point c); this energy could be achieved by feeding a formula contain 85 kcal per 100 ml at 183 ml/kg per day (point f) but it could not be achieved by feeding formulas containing only 75 or 65 kcal/dl.

Example 2

Suppose a baby can tolerate only 130 ml/kg of fluid (point g). If a formula containing 85 kcal per 100 ml is given this will provide the lower recommended amount of energy (110 kcal per 100 ml; point h). If this formula contains only the minimum recommended protein content, however (i.e. 2.25 g per 100 kcal; point j), the point is outside the box because the protein intake will be only 2.5 g/kg which is below the minimum guideline of 2.9 g/kg. To achieve the minimum guideline for protein intake a formula containing 85 kcal per 100 ml fed at 130 kcal/kg should also contain a little over 2.6 g per 100 kcal (point k).

Fat (Fig. 17.3)

There are similar, but simpler, considerations for fat. A formula containing the maximum amount of fat (7 g per 100 kcal) should not be fed to provide more than the suggested average energy intake of 130 kcal/kg since this would exceed the guideline of not more than 9 g/kg.

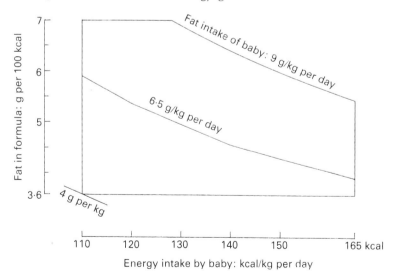

Fig. 17.3. Recommendations concerning fat: expressed as g per 100 kcal for recommended range of energy intake; also observing the maximum intake when expressed as g per kg body weight.

Carbohydrate (Fig. 17.4)

Here the limitations must be looked at differently because the upper limits are also expressed per 100 ml to avoid exceeding intestinal tolerance.

Recommendations for carbohydrate (Chapter 6) are given for total carbohydrate (illustrated on the left of the figure) and for lactose (illustrated on the right of the figure). Dealing firstly with total carbohydrate the box shows the limits implied by the recommendations, i.e. a carbohydrate energy ratio of 7–14 g per 100 kcal, an energy density in a formula of 65–85 kcal/dl and a carbohydrate concentration in the formula of not more than 11 g/dl. The lower part of the figure indicates how a formula with a particular energy density can be used to achieve varying energy intakes by the baby.

The same relationships are illustrated for lactose showing the limitations of 3.2–12 g per 100 kcal and not more than 8 g per 100 ml in a formula.

Example 1

Suppose the only carbohydrate in a formula is lactose. The formula contains 10.7 g lactose per 100 kcal. In order not to exceed the maximum recommended lactose concentration of 8 g per dl the energy density of the formula should be no more than 75 kcal per 100 ml (point a). If a formula containing 75 kcal/dl is fed to the baby a fluid intake of 147 ml/kg per day would provide the minimum recommended energy intake of 110 kcal/kg (point b); a fluid intake of 173 ml/kg would provide the average recommended energy intake of 130 kcal/kg (point c).

Example 2

Suppose a formula contained 6 g per 100 kcal of lactose and 7.5 g per 100 kcal of maltodextrin. The total carbohydrate of 13.5 g per 100 kcal remains within the guidelines. At this level of carbohydrate the energy density of the formula should not exceed 81 kcal per 100 ml otherwise the maximum recommended concentration of total carbohydrate (11 g/dl) would be exceeded (point d). At 81 kcal per 100 ml the concentration would be total carbohydrate : 10.9 g/dl; lactose 5.1 g/dl.

Example 3

Suppose a formula contained lactose 10.7 g per 100 kcal (as in Example 1) and also 2.8 g per 100 kcal of maltodextrin. The total carbohydrate of 13.5 g per 100 kcal remains within the guidelines (as in Example 2), but the energy density of the formula should not be more than 75 kcal/dl otherwise the maximum recommended concentration of lactose would be exceeded (as in Example 1). At 75 kcal/dl the calculated concentrations would be total carbohydrate: 10.1 g/dl; lactose 8.0 g/dl.

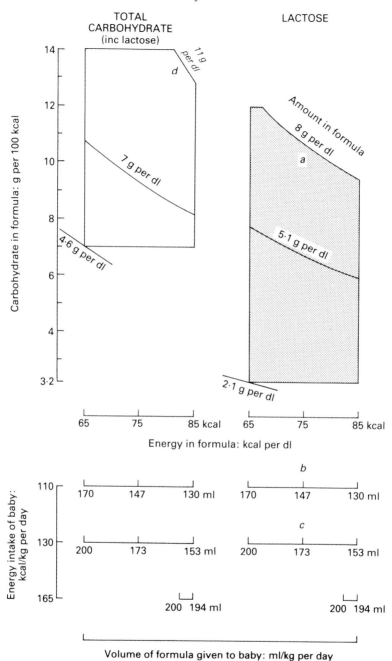

Fig. 17.4. Recommendations concerning total carbohydrate and lactose: expressed as g per 100 kcal for recommended range of energy density in a formula; also observing the maximum concentration when expressed as g per dl of formula.

Electrolytes (Fig. 17.5)

The definitive guidelines are expressed per unit volume (Chapter 7) because of their close involvement with water balance and renal solute load. There are also guidelines concerning the minimum intake by the baby (per kg body weight) and the minimum electrolyte energy ratio in a formula (mmol per 100 kcal).

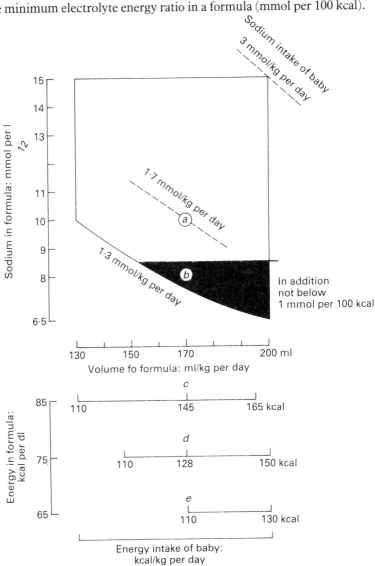

Fig. 17.5. Recommendations concerning sodium: expressed as mmol per l for the recommended range of fluid intake; also observing the recommended minimum intake by the baby (as g per kg per day) and minimum sodium energy ratio in a formula (as mmol per 100 kcal).

Using sodium as an example, the figure is again in two parts. In the upper part of the figure the four sided box indicates the limits set by the guidelines, i.e. a sodium concentration of 6.5–15 mmol/l, a fluid intake of 130–200 ml/kg per day, and a sodium intake by the baby of at least 1.3 mmol/kg per day. In addition, the concentration in a formula should not fall below 1 mmol per kcal; therefore, in the shaded area an extra check is necessary to determine that the formula meets this guideline. Above the shaded area the concentration of sodium in a formula will always exceed 1 mmol per 100 kcal.

The lower part of the figure indicates how a particular volume of intake can result in varying energy ontakes depending on the energy density of the formula.

Example 1

Suppose a formula containing 10 mmol/l is fed at 170 ml/kg per day (point a). This will achieve a sodium intake by the baby of 1.7 mmol/kg, i.e. comfortably above the minimum recommended of 1.3 mmol/kg per day. This volume of formula could achieve an energy intake between 145 kcal/kg per day (point c) and 111 kcal/kg per day (point e). Point (a) is not within the shaded area, i.e. any formula used would have a concentration greater than 1 mmol per 100 kcal (in fact varying from 1.2 mmol per 100 kcal in a formula containing 85 kcal/dl to 1.5 mmol per 100 kcal in a formula containing 65 kcal/dl).

Example 2

Suppose a formula containing 8 mmol/l is also fed at 170 ml/kg (point b). The sodium intake is again above the recommended minimum of 1.3 mmol/kg per day. Point (b) is within the shaded area, however, and, therefore, the additional check is necessary. The sodium energy ratio in a formula should not fall below 1.0 mmol per 100 kcal; use of a formula containing 8 mmol/l and 85 kcal/dl (i.e. 0.9 mmol per 100 kcal) would not meet this guideline. Formulas containing 75 and 65 kcal per dl would continue to meet that guideline, however, and they could be fed as in Example 1 to provide between 128 kcal (point d) and 111 kcal/kg per day (point e).

The figure also indicates that the maximum sodium intake *from a formula is 3 mmol/kg*. This is an important point. The limits per unit energy are from 1.0 mmol per 100 kcal (stated guideline) to 2.3 mmol per 100 kcal (*calculated* from 15 mmol/l and 65 kcal/dl). However, if a formula containing the maximum sodium: energy ratio (2.3 mmol per 100 kcal) is given this implies the use of a formula containing 65 kcal per 100 ml. The maximum energy intake achievable from such a formula is 130 kcal/kg per day, and therefore, a maximum intake of 3 mmol/kg per day (2.3 mmol per 100 kcal multiplied by

130 kcal/kg per day). It would be incorrect and (as Fig. 17.5 shows) *not* in keeping with the guidelines to take the maximum sodium energy ratio (2.3 mmol per 100 kcal) and the maximum energy intake (165 kcal/kg per day) to give a sodium intake from formula of 3.8 mmol/kg per day.

Similar considerations apply to potassium and chloride. These considerations are not illustrated but the numbers are shown in the table.

Calcium and phosphorus (Fig. 17.6)

Calcium and phosphorus each have their own individual limits and in addition a ratio limit one to each other.

Example: a formula containing 90 mg calcium and 80 mg of phosphorus per 100 kcal (point a) would meet the individual limits for each element but it is outside the box because it does not meet the guideline of a calcium phosphorus ratio of 1.4–2.0 (mg:mg). At a calcium concentration of 90 mg per 100 kcal the recommended range of phosphorus is from 64 mg (point (b); Ca:P ratio 1.4) to 50 mg (point (c) Ca:P ratio 1.8).

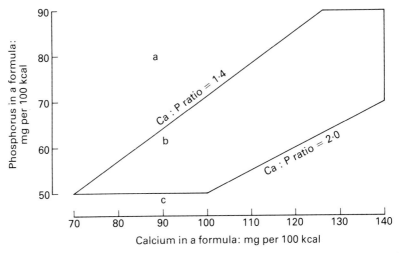

Fig. 17.6. Recommendations concerning calcium and phosphorus: expressed as mg per 100 kcal in a formula.

PRESENTATION OF THE FORMULA

Most formulas available for preterm babies are 'ready to feed', i.e. already up by the manufacturer to a predetermined concentration. This has three main advantages, ease of use, accurate composition and sterility. On the other hand, there are disadvantages. The energy and nutrient concentrations are determined by the manufacturer and cannot be increased; presentation as a concentrated liquid for dilution or as a powder for reconstitution allow feeds of varying concentration to be prepared. Ready to feed preparations are more susceptible to heat treatment (see below). Finally, ready to feed preparations are necessarily more bulky than either concentrated liquids and powder and so are less convenient for transporting home.

Ideally a formula should be available both as ready to feed (i.e. with a fixed concentration of energy and nutrients determined by the manufacturer) and as a powder or concentrated liquid suitable for mixing with water (i.e. to allow variable concentrations of energy and nutrients as determined by the paediatrician).

LABELLING

It is not the role of this Committee to give detailed labelling recommendations. Labelling concerning foods generally has been considered by many national and international bodies (1). *In addition* to any general regulations concerning the labelling of foodstuffs, however, we consider that formulas for preterm babies should carry the following information or statements on their labels:

1   A warning to the effect 'this product is intended only for preterm or low birth weight babies. It should be used only when recommended by a paediatrician and only under medical supervision'.

2   If not ready to feed then instructions for reconstitution should be given in a clear and accurate way, e.g. weight of powder to be made up to a final volume of formula, or weight of powder to be added to a volume of water to give a final volume of formula. We do not recommend the use of 'scoops' for making up these formulas but if one is supplied then the weight of powder it contains should be stated.

3   The nutrient content of the feed as given to the baby (whether as a 'ready to feed' formula or following reconstitution with water) should be stated per unit volume and per 100 kcal.

4   Instructions concerning limitations on use should be given (e.g. maximum recommended intake).

5   Reference should be made to a more detailed description of the product and its use, available from the manufacturer.

ADDITIVES and CONTAMINANTS

A number of substances may be added to a formula for 'technological reasons' such as to improve stability, etc., particularly in ready to feed formulas; examples are carrageenan and lecithin. Others are added to fortify it, e.g. iron salts. Apart from these *additives* ('intentional additives') other substances may appear in a formula as a *contaminent* ('unintentional additives') originating either from the basic raw materials, e.g. aflatoxins, chlorinated hydrocarbons, radionuclides, or during the process of manufacture and storage, e.g. lead.

We are unaware of any work concerning the effects of additives and contaminents on specifically the preterm animal. In the absence of more specific information, it seems that the recommendations applying to food generally and infant formula in particular, should be applied to formulas specifically designed for preterm babies.

In 1972 WHO commented on additives in baby foods (2) stressing the potential vulnerability of very young infants. More recently the European Community (3) and Codex Alimentarious(4) have published recommendations which include comments on additives.

HEAT TREATMENT

Heat treatment during the processing of a formula either by the manufacturer or following reconstitution in hospital, may induce a number of chemical changes. The same changes may also occur during the heat treatment of human milk. Various methods of heat treatment have been employed. Mild heat treatment will control vegetative pathogens but in the preparation of liquid ready to feed formulas exposure to higher temperatures is necessary to ensure freedom from pathogenic spores. No member of the Committee has any experience of food technology but we have considered some points concerned with heat treatment, particularly where clinical concern has been expressed.

Vitamins

Heat, especially repeated episodes of heating, may lead to partial destruction of vitamins, particularly the water soluble ones and particularly when oxygen is present during the process or on storage (5). It is usually easy to allow for this partial destruction by including a comfortable, but safe, excess over requirements in the formula. We understand that ultra high temperature processing has much less effect on vitamin content than the other heat treatments which kill spores. This process is used in the preparation of infant formulas in some, but not all, European countries. Following the reconstitution of a formula from powder a terminal sterilization or pasteurization process is performed in some hospitals. This repeated heat treatment may lead to a variable destruction of vitamins and an adequate supply from other sources, such as vitamin syrups must be ensured.

Production of lactulose

Lactulose may be found in small concentrations in ready to feed formulas (6). This has led to episodes of diarrhoea and the gut of preterm babies has an enhanced permeability to this and other macro-molecules during the first week of life (7). Adequate quality control of the heat treatment will usually prevent troublesome diarrhoea.

Protein

Three effects of heat on milk protein have attracted clinical attention, the Maillard reaction, the production of lysino alanine, and the modification of protein allergenicity.

Maillard reaction

Maillard reactions comprise the chemical reactions between carbohydrates and amino acids, for example the reactions between lactose or glucose and lysine. First N -deoxylactulosyl-lysine ('lactose-lysine') (or N -(1-deoxyfructosyl)-lysine ('fructose-lysine') are formed ('early Maillard' products) (8). By further degradation, condensation and polymerization these 'early Maillard' products are transformed to several 'advanced Maillard' products.

Measurements of lactose-lysine in commercially available lactose-containing infant formulae in Europe amounts to 3–20% of lysine (9). Because there is no method for estimating 'advanced Maillard' products, these are minimum values of blocked lysine. Storage of these formulas under inadequate conditions may increase the lysine loss still more, e.g. there is 36% loss at 60°, within 6 weeks or of 100% at 70° (10). In formulas containing monosaccharides and in lactase-treated spray-dried milk the lysine blockage can be above 50% and even with very careful processing conditions it is scarcely possible to reduce it below 15% (8). These compounds are no longer nutritionally available and their formation even with modern processing techniques cannot be prevented (11). In addition, these compounds can induce cytomegaly in rats similar to that seen with lysinoalanine (10,12).

It is impossible to give firm guidelines concerning minimum levels of *available* lysine. Total lysine in milks and formulas per 16 g N (i.e. per 100 g 'protein') are as follows

Breast milk: 5.4 g; demineralized whey 60:40 formula: 8.1 g;

Unmodified cow's milk protein 20:80 formula: 7.2 g.

Therefore, if up to 33% of lysine in a demineralized whey formula or up to 25% of the lysine in an unmodified protein formula were blocked the protein would still provide as much available lysine as a similar amount of breast milk protein.

Similarly, it is impossible to quote maximum permitted levels of fructose-lysine, but even if a formula containing the maximum recommended amount of protein (2.6 g protein, and therefore 211 mg of total lysine per 100 ml) had 20% lysine blockage by the Maillard reaction the content of lysine as fructose lysine would be considerably below that which has been observed to induce tubular cytomegaly in mature rats.

Production of lysinoalanine

Lysinoalanine is produced during sterilization of formulas. Up to 1 mg/g of crude protein may be produced by conventional sterilization (13,14). In rats lysinoalanine may induce renal cytomegaly (increase in the volume of both nucleus and cytoplasm of cells of the straight portion of the proximal tubule) which is caused by polyploidy of these cells.

The significance to infant nutrition of lysinoalanine formation in formulas and the development of renal cytomegaly in rats is not clear. No long term adverse effects have been observed in animals but no preterm or infant animals have been studied. It is, therefore, not possible to give any guidelines on maximum permitted levels in infant formulas. However, the maximum amount of lysinoalanine produced by conventional sterilization of a formula containing our maximum recommended amount of protein appears to be considerably below that which induces cytomegaly in rats (15).

General reviews of the effect of heat on nutritional quality of proteins in milk and other foods are available (16,17).

Protein allergenicity

Animal experiments suggest that β-lactoglobulin is more antigenic than either casein or the small amount of $\propto$-lactalbumin found in cow's milk (18). Compiled data from five studies of cow's milk protein intolerance in infancy showed sensitivity to β-lactoglobulin in 82%, casein in 43%, $\propto$-lactalbumin in 41%, bovine serum globulin in 27% and bovine serum albumin in 18% (19).

The use of demineralized whey formulas may, therefore, increase the intake of potential antigen. In practice this does not have any obvious ill effect. Demineralized whey formulas have been increasingly used in recent years without any obvious increase in the prevalence of cow's milk protein intolerance.

Animal and *in vitro* observations support this clinical evidence. In a series of experiments in Cambridge, the cow's milk protein sensitivity of guinea-pigs drinking different preparations of cow's milk and infant formulas was determined by the incidence of passive cutaneous anaphylaxis and the occurrence of generalized anaphylaxis following intravenous challenge with β-lactoglobulin or casein. Generally anaphylaxis to β-lactoglobulin was less common and less severe than to casein. A demineralized whey formula which contained relatively large amounts of β-lactoglobulin caused less sensitivity to both β-lactoglobulin and casein than a substituted fat formula which contained mainly casein, and a liquid concentrate of the demineralized whey formula caused even less sensitivity (20). These observations can be added to those of Saerstein *et al.* (21) who used *in vitro* precipitation and passive cutaneous anaphylaxis, and found that the antigenicity of casein β-lactoglobulin and ∝-lactalbumin was considerably reduced by current commerical milk processing. Evaporation has more effect than spray-drying, and drying more effect than pasteurization (20,21). These differential observations presumably reflect the effect of heat in reducing the potential allergenicity of β-lactoglobulin more than that of casein. Heat processing causes a number of changes in milk including the breakage of disulphide bonds. Casein is relatively heat stable up to boiling point. β-lactoglobulin has intermediate heat stability while ∝-lactalbumin is very heat labile; its antigenicity is altered by pasteurization and almost completely destroyed by procedures used in preparation of infant formulas (22,23). It could be that the reduction in allergenicity following heat treatment is insufficient to prevent allergic disease in the genetically susceptible while the reduction is of little importance to those who are not susceptible. To summarize, the potential allergenicity of cow's milk protein, as indicated by *in vitro* and animal observations, is reduced by the processes used in the manufacture of infant formulas. It is uncertain whether this reduction is on the one hand of value to the majority of infants or on the other hand sufficient for the minority with genetic susceptibility (24).

GUIDELINES

Preterm babies may receive 150–200 ml/kg per day (occasionally as low as 130 ml/kg per day) of a preterm formula containing 65–85 kcal per 100 ml to provide 110–165 kcal/kg per day.

The nutrient composition of the formula and other limitations are summarized in Table 17.1 but reference to the individual chapters is recommended for detailed considerations.

The formula should be available both 'ready to feed' at a fixed concentration and as a powder or concentrated liquid for reconstitution with water to varying concentrations.

In addition to general regulations concerning labelling of all foodstuffs, we recommend that extra information should appear on the label concerning (i) use under paediatric supervision; (ii) methods for accurate reconstitution if not ready to feed; (iii) nutrient composition; (iv) limitations on use; (v) sources of extra information.

Specific recommendations concerning heat treatment and additives and contaminants are not given. We urge manufacturers and the various national and international review bodies to keep the matter under constant review, particularly as little toxicological work has been performed in preterm mammals.

REFERENCES

1. Council Directive on the approximation of the laws of the Member States relating to the labelling, presentation, and advertising of foodstuffs for sale to the ultimate consumer (1979). *Off. J. Eur. Comm.* **L33**, 1–14.
2. FAO/WHO Expert Committee (1972). Evaluation of food additives. *WHO Technical Report Series* **488**, 28–34.
3. Astier-Dumas M., Fernandes J., Marquardt P., Mariani P., Nordio S. Oppe T.E., Schmidt E., Senterre J. & Wharton B.A. (1983). First report of the Scientific Committee for food on the essential requirements of infant formulae and follow up milks based on cows milk proteins. *Food Science and Techniques*. Reports of the Scientific Committee for Food 14 Series. Commission of the European Committees, Luxemburg 1983; EUR 8752EN: 9–32.
4. Codex Alimentarius Commission (1976). Recommended international standards for foods for infants and children. 1–33. FAO/WHO Food Standards Programme, Rome.
5. Burton H., Ford J.E., Franklin J.G. & Porter J.W.G. (1976). Effect of repeated heat treatment on the levels of some vitamins of the B complex. *J. Dairy Sci.* **34**, 193–7.
6. Bernhardt F.W., Galiardi E.D., Tomarell R.M. & Stribley R.C. (1964). Lactulose in modified milk products for infant nutrition. *J. Dairy Sci.* **48**, 399–400.
7. Beach R.O., Menzies I.S., Clayden G.S. & Scopes J.W. (1982). Gastrointestinal permeability changes in the preterm neonate. *Arch. Dis. Child.* **57**, 141–5.
8. Kaufmann W. ed. (1983). *Role of Milk Proteins in Human Nutrition*. Th. Man Publ., Gelsenkirchen-Buer. pp 301–309 and 357–368.
9. Bremer H.J., Schilling E. & Laryea M. Lysine blockage in commercially available lactose-containing infant formulae. Unpub. results.
10. Hurrell R.F., Finot P.A. & Ford J.E. (1983). Storage of milk powders under adverse conditions. 1. Losses of lysine and of other essential amino acids as determined by chemical and microbiological methods. *Br. J. Nutr.* **49**, 343–54.
11. Finot F.A., Deutsch R. & Bijard E. (1981). The extent of the Maillard reaction during the processing of milk. *Progr. Food Nutr. Sci.* **5**, 345–55.
12. Von Wangenheim B., Hanichen T. & Erbersdobler H. (1984). Histopathologische Untersuchungen an Rattennieren nach Fütterung hitzegeschädigter Proteine. *Z. Ernährungswiss* **23**, 219–29.
13. Hurrell R.F. & Carpenter K.J. (1981). The estimation of available lysine in foodstuffs after Maillard reactions. *Progr. Food Nutr. Sci.* **5**, 159–76.
14. Finot P.A. (1984). Maillard reaction products formed during processing and storage. Proc. Sem. 'Challenge to Contemporary Dairy Analytical Techniques'. Reading, England. March 28–30, 1984. International Dairy Federation.
15. Finot P.A. (1983). Lysinoalanine in food proteins. *Rev. Clin. Nutr.* **53**, 67–80.
16. Carpenter K.J. & Booth V.H. (1973). Damage to lysine in food processing: its measurement and its significance. *Nutr. Abst. Rev.* **43**, 424–49.
17. Eriksson C. (1981). Maillard reactions in Food: chemical, physiological and technological aspects. *Prog. Food Nutritr. Sci.* **5**, 1–497.
18. Ratner B., Dworetzky M., Oguri S. & Ascheim L. (1958). Studies on the allerginicity of cow's milk. 1. The allergenic properties of alpha casein, beta lactoglobulin and alpha lactalbumin. *Paediatrics* **22**, 449–52.
19. Lenethal E. (1975). Cows milk protein allergy. *Pediatr. Clin. N. Am.* **22**, 827–33.

20. Anderson K.J., McLaughlan P., Devey M.E. & Coombs R.R.A. (1979). Anaphylactic sensitivity of guinea-pigs drinking different preparations of cows milk and infant formulae. *Clin. Exp. Immunol.* **35**, 454–61.
21. Saperstein S. & Anderson D.W. (1962). Antigenicity of milk proteins. *J. Pediatr.* **61**, 196–204.
22. Ratner B., Dworetzky M., Oguri S. & Ascheim L. (1958). Studies of the allergenicity of cows milk II: Effect of heat treatment on the allergenicity of milk and protein fractions from milk as tested in guinea-pigs by parenteral sensitisation and challenge. *Pediatrics* **22**, 648–59.
23. Davies W. (1958). Cows milk allergy in infancy. *Arch. Dis. Child.* **33**, 265–8.
24. Wharton B.A. (1981). Immunological implications of alternatives to mothers milk: I. Infant Formulas. In: *The Immunology of Infant Feeding.* (ed. A.W. Wilkinson), pp 107–22. Plenum, New York.

Table 17.1. Composition of infant formula and intakes of nutrients by the baby according to stated guidelines.

Nutrients:	Nutrient per 100 kcal	Other guidelines	Concentration of nutrient per 100ml according to energy density of formula kcal/100ml			Intake per kg body weight if formula fed to provide energy intake of (kcal per kg)		
			65	75	85	110	130	165
Proximates and electrolytes								
Protein g total casein/whey (taurine)	2.25–3.1		1.5–2.0	1.7–2.3	1.9–2.6	2.9[a]–3.4	2.9–4.0[b]	3.5–4.0[b]
Fat g total	3.6–7.0		2.3–4.6	2.7–5.2	3.1–5.9	4.0–7.7	4.7–9.0[b]	5.9–9.0[b]
MCT[c]	0–2.8	Up to 40% of fatty acid	<0.9 <1.8	<1 <2	<1.2 <2.3	<1.6 <3.0	<1.8 <3.6	<2.3 <3.6
linoleic acid g lower[c]	≥0.5	at least 4.5% of energy	≥0.33	≥0.38	≥0.43	≥0.6	≥0.7	≥0.8
upper[c]	<1.4	not more than	0.4 <0.9	<0.5 <1.0	<0.6 <1.1	<0.8 <1.5	<0.9 <1.8	<1.1 <1.8
(Carnitine) (Cholesterol) (Choline)								
Carbohydrate g total	7–14		4.6–9.1	5.3–10.5	6–11[b]	7.7–15.4	9.1–18.2	11.6–22.0
lactose	3.2–12		2.1–7.8	2.4–8[b]	2.7–8[b]	3.0–13.2	4.2–16.0	5.3–16.0
Sodium[d] AW = 23 mg	23–53		15–35	17–35	20–35	30–60	30–69	30–69
mmol	1.0–2.3		0.65–1.5[d]	0.75[a]–1.5[d]	0.85[a]–1.5[d]	1.3[a]–2.6[d]	1.3[a]–3.0[d]	1.3[a]–3.0[d]
Potassium 39 mg	70–148		59–98	59–98	59–98	78–168	90–195	113–195
mmol	1.8–3.8		1.5–2.5	1.5–2.5	1.5–2.5	2.0–4.3	2.3–5.0	2.9–5.0[b]
Chloride 35 mg	46–88		39–56	39–56	39–56	49–95	60–112	74–112
mmol	1.3–2.5		1.1–1.6	1.1–1.6	1.1–1.6	1.4–2.7	1.7–3.2	2.1–3.2[b]

Table 17.1 (*Contd.*)

Nutrients:		Nutrient per 100 kcal	Other guidelines	Concentration of nutrient per 100ml according to energy density of formula kcal/100ml			Intake per kg body weight if formula fed to provide energy intake of (kcal per kg)		
				65	75	85	110	130	165
Minerals									
Calcium[e]	mg	70–140		46–92	53–105	60–119	77–154	91–182	116–231
AW = 40	mmol	1.8–3.5		1.2–2.3	1.3–2.6	1.5–3.0	1.9–3.9	2.3–4.6	2.9–5.8
Phosphorus[e]	mg	50–90		33–59	38–68	43–77	55–99	65–117	83–149
31	mmol	1.6–2.9		1.1–1.9	1.2–2.2	1.4–2.5	1.8–3.2	2.1–3.8	2.7–4.8
Calcium: Phosphorus (mg) ratio		1.4–2.0							
Magnesium	mg	6–12		3.9–7.8	4.5–9.0	5.1–10.2	6.6–13.2	7.8–15.6	9.9–19.8
24	mmol	0.25–0.5		0.16–0.32	0.19–0.37	0.27–0.42	0.28–0.55	0.33–0.65	0.41–0.82
Iron[f]	mg	approx 1.5		~1.0	~1.1	~1.3	~1.7	~2.0	~2.5
56	mmol			0.02	0.02	0.02	0.03	0.04	0.04
Copper	µg	90–120	Re evaluation may be necessary	58–78	68–90	77–102	99–132	117–156	148–198
64	µmol	1.4–1.9		0.9–1.2	1.1–1.4	1.2–1.6	1.5–2.1	1.8–2.4	2.3–3.1
Zinc	µg	550–1100		358–715	413–825	468–935	605–1210	715–1430	908–1815
65	µmol	8.5–16.9		5.5–11	6.4–12.7	7.2–14.4	9.3–18.6	11–22	14–28
Manganese	µg	2.1–8		1.4–5.2	1.6–6	1.8–6.8	2.3–8.8	2.7–10.4	3.5–13.2
55	µmol	0.04–0.15		0.03–0.09	0.03–0.11	0.03–0.12	0.04–0.16	0.05–0.19	0.06–0.24
Iodine	µg	10–45		6.5–29	7.5–34	8.5–38	11–49.5	13–58.5	16.5–74
127	µmol	0.08–0.35		0.05–0.23	0.06–0.28	0.07–0.29	0.09–0.39	0.10–0.46	0.13–0.58
(Selenium, Fluoride, Chromium, Molybdenum)			See text						

Table 17.1 (*Contd.*)

Nutrients:		Nutrient per 100 kcal	Other guidelines	Concentration of nutrient per 100ml according to energy density of formula kcal/100ml			Intake per kg body weight if formula fed to provide energy intake of (kcal per kg)		
				65	75	85	110	130	165
Vitamins									
Retinol	μg	90–150		59–98	68–113	77–128	99–165	117–195	149–248
Vitamin D[9]	μg	–3[9]	20–50 per day	–2.0	–2.2	–2.6	–3.3	–3.9	–5.0
∝ tocopherol	μg	≥600	≥900 per g of polyunsaturated fatty acids. No upper limit but see text.	≥390	≥450	≥510	≥660	≥780	≥960
Vitamin k	μg	<u>4–15</u>	See text re excessive dose	2.6–9.8	3–11.3	3.4–12.8	4.4–16.5	5.2–19.5	6.6–24.8
Thiamin	μg	<u>20–250</u>[h]		13–163	15–188	17–213	22–275	26–325	33–413
Riboflavine	μg	<u>60–600</u>[h]		39–390	45–450	57–510	66–660	78–780	99–990
Niacin equivalents	μg	<u>0.8–5</u>[h]	≥800 μg niacin/100 kcal	0.5–3.3	0.6–3.8	0.7–4.3	0.9–5.5	1.0–6.5	1.3–8.3
B$_6$	μg	<u>35–250</u>[h]	≥15μg/g protein	23–163	26–188	30–213	39–275	46–325	58–413
B$_{12}$	μg	<u>≥0.15</u>		≥0.10	≥0.11	≥0.13	≥0.17	≥0.2	≥0.25
Folic acid	μg	<u>≥60</u>	at least 65 per day	≥39	≥45	≥51	≥66	≥78	≥99
Pantothenic acid	μg	<u>≥300</u>		≥195	≥225	≥255	≥330	≥390	≥495
Biotin	μg	<u>≥1.5</u>		≥1.0	≥1.1	≥1.3	≥1.7	≥2.0	≥2.5
(Inositol)	(mg)								
Vitamin C	mg	7.5–40[h]		4.9–26	5.6–30	6.4–34	8.3–44	9.8–52	12.4–66

Notes to Table 17.1.

The definitive guidelines are underlined. Other figures are obtained by calculation from these guidelines.

a   limit by calculation is lower, but figure is the lowest recommended in the guidlines

b   limit by calculation is higher, but the figure given is the highest recommended in the guidelines

c   calculations are correct to first decimal point (i.e. to nearest 0.1) but where guideline is "not less than" or "nor more than" calculation is rounded down or up respectively

d   extra sodium may be added according to individual indications

e   must also conform to guideline for calcium phosphorus ratio

f   if formula aims to provide all iron requirements

g   Vitamin D content must be clearly labelled

h   upper limit for vitamin is not a firm recommendation and is based solely on the amounts found in presently available formulas

AW: Atomic weight of element

Nutrients shown in parentheses are discussed in earlier chapters but firm quantative guidelines are not given

Index

229